Medical Terms for Nurses

A QUICK REFERENCE GUIDE

Second Edition

Janet Duffey
RN, MS, APRN, BC

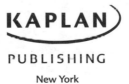

PUBLISHING

New York

© 2009 by Kaplan, Inc.

Published by Kaplan Publishing,
a division of Kaplan, Inc.
1 Liberty Plaza, 24th Floor
New York, NY 10006

Printed in the United States of America

10   9   8   7   6   5   4   3   2

ISBN-13: 978-1-60714-048-1

Kaplan Publishing books are available at special quantity discounts to use for sales promotions, employee premiums, or educational purposes. Please email our Special Sales Department to order or for more information at kaplanpublishing@kaplan.com, or write to Kaplan Publishing, 1 Liberty Plaza, 24th Floor, NY, NY 10006.

Contents

Introduction

➤ **HOW TO USE THIS BOOK**

Medical terms are the common language of many health disciplines, including medicine, nursing, physical therapy, social work, and other ancillary health care disciplines. Regardless of the discipline, it is imperative that health professionals use medical terms in a manner that reflects knowledge and efficiency. This book was created for use by teachers, students, and experienced clinicians alike to enhance and to increase their medical term vocabulary.

It is important to note that considerable variation exists in how nurses learn medical terminology in their academic course work. Some schools require a separate medical terminology class, while others use an integrated approach throughout their curriculum. Notwithstanding the debate on how to best prepare nurses for the challenges of clinical practice, the task of mastering ever-evolving medical innovation and associated language is a challenge for all. This resource will attempt to fill the void between initial educational preparation and the realities of constant change and innovation in clinical practice.

Included in the introduction of this book is an explanation of how medical terms are formed. This foundation is the basis for understanding the approximately 3,400 medical terms contained herein, and will provide you with an effective method of increasing your professional vocabulary throughout your career. While it may be tempting to jump to the alphabetized list for a definition, this section also covers the basic elements of medical terms: prefixes, roots, and suffixes.

The 3,400 terms found in Section 1 have been selected for their accuracy and relevance to multiple patients and practice settings; no single practice area or setting has been deliberately excluded. The terms, including prefixes, suffixes, and roots, are listed alphabetically for convenience. Each term is followed by a phonetic pronunciation and brief definition, but plural forms and synonyms are included only when appropriate. Please note that the definitions provided assume some prior knowledge of anatomy, physiology, and pathological or disease states. It is a supplement to knowledge, but not a full-length pathophysiology text.

In the second section of this book, selected terms are categorized in resource lists based on anatomy, pathologies or diseases, and procedures. Diagrams have also been included to clarify structures related to some anatomical terms. The final resource list is a collection of the most common prefixes, word roots, and suffixes. This may well offer the greatest utility in deciphering the numerous permutations of medical conditions, diagnostics, and interventions in the practice of nursing and related disciplines.

Finally, in Section 3 you will find a comprehensive list of common medical abbreviations. Not all have been covered within the 3,400 terms, so you should use this as a supplemental resource.

➤ HOW MEDICAL WORDS ARE FORMED

Most medical words are comprised of four basic elements:

- word roots
- combining forms
- prefixes
- suffixes

While not all words are comprised of all four parts, most have at least two. By analyzing and determining the individual meanings of these parts, the total meaning can be derived even when you are not familiar with the exact word. This approach removes the need for endless memorization of terms in relative isolation one from another.

Each of these four elements is discussed in greater detail here.

Word Roots

A word root is similar to a subject of a sentence. Often derived from Latin or Greek, it defines the main topic or feature of the word. Typically, the root is in the middle, preceded by a prefix and followed by a variation called a combining form and a suffix—more on these later. A root is essential to the subject of the word. Finding the root is the first clue in deciphering multipart medical terms.

Some roots stand alone. For example, *bruit*, *prostate*, *fever*, *alcohol*, and *thyroid* can be used alone, but are more specific when combined with prefixes or suffixes.

Example:
Tendon is the root in the term *tendonitis*. By combining the root with the suffix *-itis*, we add the meaning of "inflammation of the tendon." Therefore, the translation of the term *tendonitis* is reliant on the root term being modified or described by the suffix.

Prefixes

Prefixes are highly descriptive word parts at the beginning of the term that lend a specific context to the term. A small selection of commonly used prefixes include: *pre-* (before), *post-* (after), *ab-* (move away from center), *ad-* (move toward center), and *pseudo-* (false or similar to).

Common classifications of prefixes include:

- number (e.g., *bi-* meaning two, *quad-* meaning four)
- size (e.g., *mega-* meaning large, *micro-* meaning small)
- directional (e.g., *para-* meaning beside, *ab-* meaning toward the midline)
- organ (e.g., *encephal-* meaning brain, *hepat-* meaning liver)
- quality (e.g., *dys-* meaning painful, difficult, or bad; *neo-* meaning new)

Example:
Pseud- is the prefix in the term *pseudodementia*. By combining *pseud-* with the root *dementia* and using the combining form "o," we create the meaning of "false decreased cognitive function."

Combining Forms

Joining of prefixes, root terms, and suffixes is accomplished by using a combining vowel; usually the letter "o" to join the two word parts. Combining forms do not have a specific meaning and do not stand alone, but serve to link the two or more word elements into one word.

Example:
Endocrine means "organs secreting directly into bloodstream," and *-logy* means "the study of." The sum

meaning of the root and suffix is "the study of organs that secrete directly into the bloodstream." Replacing the "e" at the end of *endocrine* with the linking combining form "o" facilitates joining the two terms into one word with a highly descriptive meaning.

Suffixes

Located at the end of a word, suffixes modify the meaning of the word root. Within medical terms, a suffix often describes a disease, condition, structure, procedure, or treatment. Additionally, suffixes can indicate parts of speech such as nouns, adjectives, or diminutive expression.

- A noun suffix describes the condition and may be singular or plural. Examples of noun suffixes describing a condition are: *-esis*, *-ia*, and *-ism*. Noun suffixes are also used to name specific areas of clinical specialty. Examples include: *-iatry* (study or practice of a certain area) and *-ist* (specialist in a particular area).

- In their adjective form, suffixes give great meaning to the root term. Suffixes that mean "related or pertaining to" include: *-ac*, *-al*, *-ar*, *-ary*, *-eal*, *-ic*, *-ile*, *-ior*, *-ous*, and *-tic*. There is one combination suffix: *-ical*, which is a combination of *-ic* and *-al*.

- Diminutive suffixes indicate the small size or scale of the term. Examples of diminutive suffixes are: *-y*, *-icle*, *-ole*, *-ule*.

KAPLAN

Forming Medical Terms

Considerable variation exists in the ability to explain medical phenomena using prefixes, roots, and suffixes. The simplest is a stand-alone root, for example, *phobia*. Many terms include at least one prefix, root, and suffix; for example: *hyper/tens/ive*.

The use of two or more prefixes adds both specificity and complexity to the term. For example: *chol/angio/pancreato/graphy* means "the study of pancreas and bile ducts using x-rays." Terms with this level of complexity are often used to describe a multisystem condition's symptoms, or diagnostic and operative interventions.

Rules for Combining Forms

1. Word roots link a suffix beginning with a vowel.

   Example: [*append-* + *-ectomy*] becomes *appendectomy*

2. Combining forms where the suffix begins with a consonant is the root word + "o."

   Example: [*gynec* + *o*] + *mastia* = *gynecomastia* (gynec/o becomes the combining form)

3. Compound words are formed by linking two root words with "o" in the middle, even when the second root begins with a vowel.

   Example: [*oste-* + *o*] + *arthritis* = *osteoarthritis*

4. No vowel is added when the suffix begins with a vowel.

   Example: gastro- + -itis = gastritis

5. Plural forms of words are dictated by the last letter(s) of the singular form. This rule is demonstrated in the table below.

From Singular to Plural Forms

Changing a singular form to the plural form entails modification of the suffix. The following table summarizes the rules for conversion of common singular to plural suffixes. Example terms demonstrating the change from singular to plural are provided.

Singular Suffix	Plural Suffix	Rule for Conversion	Singular to Plural Examples
-a	*-ae*	Keep the "a," add "e"	scapula to scapulae
-ax	*-aces*	Remove "x," add "ces"	pneumothorax to pneumothoraces
-en	*-ina*	Remove "en," add "ina"	foramen to foramina
-ex	*-ices*	Remove "ex," add "ices"	apex to apices
-is	**-es**	Remove "is," add "es"	diagnosis to diagnoses

Singular Suffix	Plural Suffix	Rule for Conversion	Singular to Plural Examples
-ix	*-ices*	Remove "ix," add "ices"	calix to calices
-ma	*-mata* *-mas*	Keep "ma," add "ta" OR Add "s" to the end	chondroma to chondromata fibromyoma to fibromyomas
-nx	*-nges*	Remove "x," add "ges"	phalanx to phalanges
-on	*-a*	Remove "on," add "a"	ganglion to ganglia
-um	*-a*	Remove "um," add "a"	bacterium to bacteria
-us	*-i*	Remove "us," add "i"	sulcus to sulci
-y	*-ies*	Remove "y," add "ies"	biopsy to biopsies

ABCs of Quick Term Definitions

1. **A**nalyze the word parts (prefix, root, suffix)

2. **B**ring the word-part definitions into the order of: suffix, prefix, and root or combining form.

3. **C**omplete the conceptual definition by adding words to link the definitions into a descriptive phrase. For example, *gastroenteritis* would be interpreted by word parts as "stomach, small intestine, inflammation." Rearranged into logical order, it becomes: "inflammation of the stomach and small intestine."

Conclusion

By mastering the basic building blocks and a few rules, effective communication using medical terms can be used to produce quality patient care across many disciplines. When the exact definition isn't known by rote memorization, these analytic skills provide valuable clues to accurate definitions.

Glossary

ALPHABETICAL LISTING OF TERMS

17-ketosteroids test [17 kee-toh-STEER-oidz test] a 24-hour urine test to detect steroidal metabolites of androgenic and adrenocortical hormones

3-methoxy-4-hydroxymandelic acid test [3 meth-OK-see 4 high-DROK-see-man-DEL-ick as-id test] urine test to detect possible muscular dystrophy

A

a- [ah] *prefix*; without

ab- [ab] *prefix*; away from

abdominal [ab-DOM-ih-nal] pertaining to the abdomen

abdominal aorta [ab-DOM-ih-nal aye-OR-tah] major blood vessel supplying blood to the abdominal organs

abdominal hernia [ab-DOM-ih-nal HUR-nee-uh] abnormal protrusion of an organ through the abdominal musculature

abdominopelvic [ab-DOM-ih-noh-PEL-vik] pertaining to the region of the body including the abdomen, pelvis (including the renal pelvis), and hip bone

abduction [ab-DUK-shun] to draw away from

aberrant conduction [AB-er-ant kon-DUKT-shun] passage of electrical impulses of the heart through abnormal pathways

aberratio testis [ab-er-AYE-shee-oh test-eez] location of a testicle in an abnormal anatomical position

ablation [ab-LAY-shun] destruction of tissue or function by surgery, electrocautery, or radio frequency

-able [uh-bul] *suffix*; able to be

ablepharia [ab-leh-FAY-ree-ah] congenital defect of eyelid formation, eyelid is either absent or reduced in size

ablepsia [ah-BLEP-see-ah] inability to see; blindness

abrasion [ah-BRAY-zhun] wearing down of a surface, such as skin, by rubbing or scraping

abruptio placenta [ah-BRUP-shee-oh pla-SEN-tah] sudden and premature separation of the placenta from the site of uterine attachment due to bleeding between the placenta and uterine wall

abscess [AB-sess] a cavity containing pus and surrounded by inflamed tissue

absence seizure [AB-senz SEE-zur] brain dysfunction involving a brief loss of consciousness without motor involvement; also called petit-mal seizure

absorption [ab-SORP-shun] process by which digested food nutrients move through villi of the small intestine into the blood

abstinence [AB-sti-nenz] refraining from certain behaviors, activities, foods, or beverages

abstract [AB-strakt] summary statement of research article that identifies the purpose, methodology, findings, and conclusions

abulia [ah-BYOO-lee-ah] impaired ability to make decisions, perform voluntary actions, react emotionally or verbally; commonly associated with bilateral frontal lobe disease

ac- [ak] *prefix*; pertaining to

acantha [ah-KAN-tha] general term for spine, especially the spinous process of a vertebra

acanthosis [ak-an-THOH-sis] breakdown or separation of the prickle-cell layer of the epidermis leading to cellular degeneration

acataphasia [ah-kat-ah-FAY-zee-ah] an inability to choose words that accurately reflect thoughts and/or to speak correct words due to a cerebral lesion

accommodation [ah-com-moh-DAY-shun] adaptation or adjustment to physical or psychological changes; adjustment of the eye to focus on objects at various distances

acet- [as-eet] *prefix*; vinegar; acid; sour; sharp

acetabulum [as-ee-TAB-yoo-lum] a cup-shaped socket in the hip bone, formed by the ilium, that is occupied by the head of the femur, forming the hip joint

acetylcholine [as-ee-til-KOH-leen] chemical involved in nerve impulse transmission

Achilles reflex [ah-KIL-eez REE-flecks] contraction of the calf muscle following a sharp blow to the Achilles tendon behind the ankle

Achilles tendon [ah-KIL-eez TEN-don] tendon of the lower leg that extends from the gastrocnemius and soleus muscles and attaches to the calcaneus bone of the heel; it is the thickest and strongest tendon of the body

achillorrhaphy [ah-kil-OR-ah-fee] surgical repair of the Achilles tendon by suturing

acidosis [as-ih-DOH-sis] an abnormal increase in hydrogen ion concentration in the body

acne vulgaris [AK-nee vul-GAIR-ris] inflammation of the hair follicle and associated sebaceous glands

acoustic neuroma [ah-KOOS-tik nyoo-ROH-mah] benign tumor of the vestibulocochlear nerve resulting in pain, headache, hearing loss, tinnitus, and disturbed balance

acquired immunodeficiency syndrome (AIDS) [ah-kwyrd IM-yoo-noh-dee-FISH-en-see SIN-drom] syndrome of immune disruption with opportunistic diseases such as pneumonia, Kaposi's sarcoma, and others due to infection with human immunodeficiency virus by sexual contact and blood-borne exposure

acrodynia [AK-roh-din-ee-ah] a disease of infants and young children manifest by edematous skin, scarlet coloration of the face and lips, pink coloration of extremities, cold, clammy and painful skin along with generalized dia-phoresis, photophobia, and failure to thrive. Etiology is thought to be Mercury poisoning

acromegaly [ak-roh-MEG-ah-lee] excessive secretion of the growth hormone somatotropin that produces enlargement of head, face, hands, and feet

acromion [ah-KROH-mee-on] a long, bladelike spine along the upper half of the scapula bone

acrotism [ak-ROH-tizm] having an undetectable pulse

actin [AK-tin] a muscle protein that is responsible for muscle contraction

actinic keratosis [ak-TIN-ik ker-ah-TOH-sis] localized thickening and scaling of the outer layers of the skin as a result of prolonged exposure to the sun

actinotherapy [AK-tin-oh-THER-ah-pee] treatment of skin disorders using rays such as ultraviolet radiation

action potential [AK-shun poh-TEN-shul] the change in electrical charge within a nerve or muscle when stimulated

activated charcoal [AK-ti-vay-ted CHAR-kol] an agent given by mouth or nasogastric tube to absorb toxic substances in the stomach

active euthanasia [AK-tiv yoo-tha-NAY-zee-ah] process of tak-ing deliberate action that will hasten the client's death

acupressure [AK-yoo-pres-shur] use of finger pressure applied to specific nerve junctions on the body to promote healing

-acusis [ah-koo-sis] *suffix*; related to hearing

acute [ah-KYOOT] intense, sharp, severe symptoms followed by a short course of illness

acute crisis [ah-KYOOT KRI-sis] severe state of disorganization that occurs when the individual's usual coping mechanisms, physical or emotional, are no longer effective

acute pain [ah-KYOOT payn] discomfort identified by sudden onset and relatively short duration, mild to severe intensity, and a steady decrease in intensity over several days or weeks

acute respiratory distress syndrome [ah-KYOOT RES-pih-ra-tore ee dis TRES SIN-drom] massive damage to alveoli due to injury to lungs from burns, aspiration of vomitus, or infection which renders the lungs incapable of making surfactant required to keep lung tissue open

ad- [ad] *prefix*; toward midline or near

-ad [ahd] *suffix*; toward or in direction of

adaptation [ad-ap-TAY-shun] component of cognitive development that refers to the changes that occur as a result of assimilation and accommodation; ongoing process by which an individual adjusts to stressors in order to achieve homeostasis

addiction [ah-DIK-shun] a state of complete physical and psychological dependence on a substance

Addison's disease [AD-dih-suns dis-EEZ] chronic adrenocortical insufficiency possibly due to autoimmune disease, adrenal tumors, or tuberculosis

adductor longus muscle [a-DUCK tur LONG-us MUS-sel] muscle of the thigh and one of five medial femoral muscles; it functions to adduct and flex the thigh

adductor magnus muscle [a-DUCK-tur MAG-nus MUS-sel] muscle of the medial aspect of the thigh which acts to adduct the thigh; the proximal portion acts to rotate the thigh medially and to flex it on the hip

-ade [ayd] *suffix*; action or process

adenitis [ad-eh-NY-tis] inflammation of a gland or lymph node

adenocarcinoma [AD-eh-ooh-KAR-sih-NOH-mah] cancer tumor, mass gland

adenohypophysis [ad-ee-noh-high-POF-ih-sis] anterior pituitary gland, which produces hormones

adenoids [AD-en-oydz] lymphatic tissue on the back of the nasopharynx; also called pharyngeal tonsil

adenosine [ah-DEN-oh-seen] a highly potent vasodilator used to perform cardiovascular perfusion studies without having the client exercise

adenosine monophosphate [ah-DEN-oh-seen mon-oh-FOS-fayt] a hormone secreted by the parafocicular cells of the thyroid gland to regulate the level of blood calcium

adenosine triphosphate (ATP) [ah-DEN-oh-seen try-FOS-fate] a molecular substance that supplies the energy for muscle fiber contraction; energy is released when ATP is hydrolyzed to adenosine diphosphate

adenovirus [AD-eh-noh-VY-rus] a large group of viruses causing common colds and upper respiratory tract infections

adherence [ad-HEER-ents] the degree of compliance or continuance of a therapeutic action; ability of two surfaces to stick together

adhesion [ad-HEE-zhun] abnormal fibrous bands of tissue that form after abdominal or other surgeries

adipose [AD-ih-poze] fat

adipsia [ah-DIP-see-ah] lack of normal thirst

adjustment disorder [ad-JUST-ment dis-OR-der] psychiatric illness characterized by gross inability to effectively respond to a major stressful life event

adnexa [ad-NEK-sa] connecting parts of a structure; as demonstrated in the uterine adnexa, which includes the uterine tubes, ovaries, and uterine ligaments

adrenal cortex [ah-DREE-nal KOHR-tex] outer portion of the adrenal gland

adrenal glands [ah-DREE-nal glanz] endocrine gland located on each kidney; comprised of the adrenal cortex, which excretes steroid hormones, and the adrenal medulla, which secretes epinephrine and norepinephrine

adrenal medulla [ah-DREE-nal me-DEW-luh] inner portion of the adrenal gland

adrenal virilism [ah-DREE-nal VIR-ih-lizm] masculine facial and body features in females due to hypersecretion of androgens

adrenalectomy [ah-dree-nal-EK-toh-mee] surgical removal of the adrenal gland

adrenaline [ah-DREN-ah-lin] epinephrine; hormone secreted by the adrenal medulla

adrenocortical steroid hormone [ah-DREE-noh-KOR-ti-kal STEER-oyd HOR-mohn] hormones, including glucocorticoids, mineralocorticoids, and androgens, that are produced by the adrenal cortex

adrenocorticotropic hormone (ACTH) [ah-DREE-noh-kor-tih-koh-TROP-ik HOR-mohn] a hormone secreted by the pituitary gland that stimulates the release of hormones from the renal cortex

advance directive [ad-VANCE DYE-rek-tiv] written instruction for health care that is recognized under state law and is used in the provision of such care when the individual is incapacitated

adventitious breath sounds [ad-ven-TISH-us breth sownds] abnormal sounds, such as crackles and rhonchi, heard in the lungs during auscultation

adverse reaction [ad-VERS re-AK-shun] drug effect contrary to what is therapeutically intended

aer- [er] *prefix*; gas or air

aerobic metabolism [air-RO-bik me-TAB-oh-lizm] processing of nutrients in the presence of oxygen; a metabolic pathway that uses oxygen to convert glucose into cellular energy

aerocele [ER-oh-seel] distention of a bodily cavity with gas

aerocoly [er-OK-oh-lee] distention of the colon with gas

aerocystoscopy [er-oh-sis-TOS-koh-pee] visual examination of the bladder using a cystoscope while the bladder is distended by air

aerophagia [air-oh-FAY-jee-ah] swallowing air during eating or drinking liquids

affect [AF-fekt] outward display on the face

affective disorder [ah-FEK-tiv dis-OR-der] a psychiatric condition characterized by disturbance of mood; most commonly depression or anxiety

affective domain [af-FEK-tiv doe-MAIN] area of learning that involves attitudes, beliefs, and emotions

afferent [AF-fer-ent] to transport or carry toward the center; nerves that return impulses to the central nervous system

afferent lymphatic vessel [AF-fer-ent lim-FAT-ik VES-el] a small structure that transports lymph from the periphery or distal portions of the body, draining into more central vessels or lymph nodes

afferent nerve [AF-fer-ent nerv] any nerve that transmits impulses from receptors in the peripheral nervous system to the central nervous system; opposite of an efferent nerve

agglutination [ah-gluh-tih-NAY-shun] the clumping together of cells as a result of interaction with specific antibodies called agglutinins; agglutinins are used in blood tests that determine the blood type—such as A, B, AB, and O—and Rh factor (positive or negative); derived from a Latin word meaning "glue together"

aggregates [AG-gre-gates] individuals, families, and other subgroupings of people who are associated because of singular social, personal, or health care needs; a group or population

agnosia [ag-NOH-see-ah] loss of the ability to comprehend sensory input despite normal sensory function

agonist [AG-on-ist] pharmacological agent that combines with receptors to initiate drug actions

agoraphobia [AG-or-ah-FOH-bee-ah] fear of crowds or public places which causes individuals to resist leaving home even for important or urgent medical care

-agra [ag-rah] *suffix*; sudden, severe pain

agranulocytosis [aye-GRAN-yoo-loh-sigh-TOH-sis] acute, life-threatening immunocompromised state characterized by severe depression or complete absence of disease-fighting white blood cells and by leukopenia, resulting in infections of the skin and mucous membranes

agraphia [aye-GRAF-ee-ah] inability to write due to cerebral pathology

air embolism [air EM-bo-lizm] entrance of air into a blood vessel, most often a vein, during trauma or medical procedures; if the amount of air is large enough, death can result

airborne precautions [air-born pre-KAW-shuns] actions taken to stop transmission of infectious agents by exposure to airborne droplet spray, including air filtration systems and masks

air-puff tonometry [air-puff ton-OM-eh-tree] assessment of intraocular pressure using a burst of air rebounding off the cornea without the instrument touching the patient's eye

-al [ul] *suffix*; pertaining or related to

alanine aminotransferase test [AL-uh-neen ah-mee-noh-TRANS-fer-ace test] blood enzyme test to evaluate tissue damage

alarm reaction [ah-LARM ree-AK-shun] initial phase of general adaptation syndrome; bodily response to stress by release of endocrine hormones preparing for fight or flight

alb- [alb] *prefix*; white color, or lacking of normal pigments

Albert's disease [AL-bertz dis-EEZ] bursitis of the Achilles tendon with or without calcification; due to trauma or poorly fitting shoes

albinism [AL-bih-nizm] hereditary absence of melanin pigment in the body

albino [al-BI-noh] lacking pigmentation of the skin, eyes, and hair

albumin [al-BEW-min] a major protein molecule in the blood produced by the liver

albuminuria [al-bew-mi-NEW-ree-ah] abnormal presence of the protein albumin in the urine

Alcock's canal [AL-koks kah-NAL] space in the pelvis between the obturator internus muscle and the obturator fascia that the pudendal nerve passes through

alcoholic cirrhosis [al-ko-HOL-ik sir-ROH-sis] liver enlargement, fatty deposits, and fibrosis due to chronic ethanol abuse

aldosterone [al-DOS-ter-ohn] a mineralocorticoid steroid hormone that stimulates the renal tubule in the kidneys to retain water and sodium

-algia [ahl-jee-ah] *suffix*; painful condition

algophobia [al-go-FO-bee-ah] morbid or excessive fear and sensitivity to pain

algor mortis [AL-gore MOHR-tis] lack of skin elasticity as a result of death

algorithm [AL-go-rith-im] a formula or set of rules for diagnosis and treatment of a disease

alimentary canal [al-ih-MEN-tar-ee kah-NAL] gastro-intestinal system including all structures from the mouth to the anus

alimentation [al-ih-men-TAY-shun] giving of food or nourishment to the body by natural or artificial means such as feeding tubes or intravenous injection

-alis [ah-lis] *suffix*; pertaining or related to

alkaline phosphatase test [AL-kah-line FAWS-fah-tace] blood test for the enzyme alkaline phosphatase that is found in both liver cells and bone cells; elevated blood levels are suggestive of liver or bone disease

alkalosis [al-ka-LOW-sis] an abnormal condition of body fluids, characterized by a tendency toward a blood pH level greater than 7.45; this level is caused by an excess of alkaline bicarbonate or deficiency of acid

alkalosis, compensated [al-ka-LOW-sis, KOM-pen-say-ted] metabolic state where the pH of the blood has returned to normal with increased level of bicarbonate in the blood

alkalosis, hypochloremic [al-ka-LOW-sis, hy-po-klo-REE-mik] metabolic state of increased pH of the blood due to loss of chloride; associated with aggressive diuresis, severe vomiting, and drainage of gastric acid by nasogastric tube

alkalosis, hypokalemic [al-ka-LOW-sis, hy-po-ka-LEE-mik] metabolic state of increased pH of the blood due to excessive loss of potassium; often associated with diuretic therapy

alkalosis, metabolic [al-ka-LOW-sis, met-ah-BOL-ik] metabolic state where bicarbonate levels of the blood are increased resulting from loss of acid from the gastrointestinal tract or kidney, diuretic therapy, intake of alkaline foods, or adrenal gland hyperactivity

alkalosis, respiratory [al-ka-LOW-sis, RES-pih-ra-tore-ree] metabolic state where pH of the blood is increased due to hyperventilation resulting in decreased

carbon dioxide and subsequent reduction of plasma
bicarbonate levels

Allen test [AL-len test] procedure that measures the
collateral circulation to the radial artery

allergenic extract [al-er-JEN-ik EKS-trakt] protein substance
from various foods, pollens, and other sources for the
purpose of skin testing and desensitization

allergic rhinitis [ah-LER-jik rye-NIGH-tis] nasal mucous
membrane inflammation caused by allergen inhalation;
allergies may be seasonal or year-round

allo- [al-oh] *prefix*; referring to another

allodynia [AL-oh-dye-nee-uh] pain caused by a stimulus
that does not normally evoke pain

allogeneic [AL-oh-jeh-NEE-ik] bone marrow, stem cells, or
other tissue donated by another person

allograft [AL-oh-graft] frozen or freeze-dried bone taken
from a cadaver

allopathic [AL-oh-path-ik] medical treatments recognized
by a specific culture as being traditional, conventional,
or mainstream; for example, Western medicine

alopecia [al-oh-PEE-shee-ah] partial or complete lack of
hair; partial lack on scalp and face (areata); complete
lack on scalp (totalis); complete lack of any body
hair (universalis)

alpha waves [AL-fah wayvz] brain waves typical of a person
who is awake and at rest

alternative medicine [al-TER-nah-tiv MED-ih-sin] treatment
approaches that are not accepted by mainstream
Western medical practice, such as acupuncture,
chiropractics, hypnosis, etc.

alveolar hypoventilation [al-VEE-oh-lar hy-po-ven-tih-LAY-
shun] inability to fully expand and fill the small hollow
cavities of the lungs

alveoli [al-VEE-oh-lie] hollow, sphere-shaped cells of the lung
that function to exchange oxygen and carbon dioxide

Alzheimer's disease [AWL-zye-murz dis-EEZ] a degenerative brain disorder that causes dementia and physical deterioration with typical onset late in life; disrupts brain function by formation of amyloid plaques, neurofibrillary tangles, and cerebral atrophy

ambi- [am-bi] *prefix*; both or two ways

amblyopia [am-blee-OH-pee-ah] impaired vision that is unrelated to an ocular lesion and cannot be fully corrected with glasses; most likely cause is abnormal vision during developmental years

amebiasis [am-eh-BY-ah-sis] infection with *Entamoeba histolytica* that is spread by ingestion of contaminated food

amenorrhea [ah-men-oh-REE-ah] absence of menstruation

amnesia [am-NEE-zee-ah] partial or total loss of long-term memory due to trauma or disease of hippocampus

amniocentesis [AM-nee-oh-sen-TEE-sis] transabdominal needle aspiration of amniotic fluid from the amniotic sac for diagnostic purposes

amnion [AM-nee-on] a thin, transparent, internal fetal membrane that contains the amnionic fluid and fetus during pregnancy

amniorrhexis [am-nee-or-REK-sis] rupture of the amnion

amniotome [AM-nee-oh-tohm] instrument used to puncture the amnionic membrane

amniotomy [am-nee-OT-oh-mee] surgical incision of the amnion to induce labor

amphi [am-fee] *prefix*; both sides or double

amphiarthrosis [am-fee-ar-THRO-sis] a slightly moveable joint where the surfaces of the opposing bones are connected by cartilage, as seen in the symphysis pubis

amputation [am-pyoo-TAY-shun] removal of an extremity due to trauma or circulatory disease; classified as traumatic or surgical depending on the circumstances in which removal occurred

amputee [AM-pyoo-tee] an individual who has lost an extremity or phalange

amygdaloid body [ah-MIG-dah-loyd boh-DEE] an almond-shaped area of grey, unmyelinated nerve tissue located in each temporal lobe that plays a major role in processing memory and sensing dangerous situations

amyl- [am-il] *prefix*; starch

amylase [AM-ih-lays] an enzyme that breaks starch down into smaller carbohydrates; found in starch and pancreatic juice

amyotrophic lateral sclerosis (ALS) [aye-mee-oh-TROH-fik LAT-er-ahl skle-ROH-sis] an idiopathic degenerative disease of upper and lower motor neurons, causing motor weakness and spastic limbs; commonly known as Lou Gehrig's disease

an- [an] *prefix*; without, not

ana- [ah-nah] *prefix*; up or apart, excessive

anabolism [ah-NAB-oh-lizm] constructive phase of metabolism

anacusis [an-ah-KOO-sis] total deafness

anaerobic metabolism [an-er-OH-bik me-TAB-oh-lizm] a process of converting glucose into energy in the absence of oxygen

analgesia [an-al-JEE-zee-uh] condition of not experiencing any pain sensation

analyte [AN-ah-lyte] any substance that is measured, usually applied to a component of blood or other body fluid; substance dissolved in a solution; also called solute

anamnestic response [an-am-NES-tik REE-spons] immune reaction due to formation of antibodies to a pathogenic organism

anaphia [an-AH-fee-ah] inability to perceive the sensation of touch

anaphylaxis [an-uh-fil-AK-sis] extreme, immediate, hypersensitive reaction to an antigen, protein, or drug with systemic effects including bronchospasm, peripheral edema, and laryngeal edema; these effects may be life threatening

anaplasia [an-ah-PLAY-ze-ah] a term applied to cancerous cells that revert to a less developed state in arrangement and structure; a loss of differentiation among cells

anastomosis [ah-NAS-toh-MO-sis] to connect two vessels, often blood vessels or bowel segments, to allow continuous flow

anatomical position [AN ah-TOM-ih-kal poe-ZIH-shun] body positioned erect, standing, facing forward, arms at sides, palms forward, and toes pointing forward

anatomy [ah-NAT-oh-mee] study of structures of the human body

-ance [ans] *suffix*; state of

ancillary [AN-sih-lair-ee] accessory or secondary

-ancy [an-cee] *suffix*; state of

androgens [AN-droh-jinz] hormone promoting male secondary sex characteristics

anemia [ah-NEE-mee-ah] reduction in the amount of hemoglobin in the blood, thus decreasing the oxygen-carrying capacity of the blood

anesthesia [AN-es-THEE-zee-ah] pharmacological agents used to block nerve sensations

aneurysm [AN-yoo-riz-um] a localized dilation of the wall of a blood vessel

ang- [anj] *prefix*; distress, choke

angina pectoris [an-JYE-nah PECK-tor-is] chest pain that radiates to the left shoulder

angiocatheter [AN-jee-oh-KATH-eh-ter] a hollow, flexible tube inserted into a blood vessel to withdraw or instill fluids

angioedema [AN-jee-oh-eh-DEE-ma] sudden, well-defined, large area of edema often due to an allergy to foods or drugs

angiogenesis [an-jee-oh-JEN-eh-sis] formation of new blood vessels

angiogram [AN-jee-oh-gram] radiographic visualization after injecting a radiopaque contrast dye into the bloodstream, enabling the vessels to be "mapped," and identifying areas of narrowing or blockage

angioplasty [AN-jee-oh-plas-tee] surgical intervention of diseased vessels for recanalization of a blood vessel; balloon dilation, mechanical stripping, injection of fibrinolytics, or placement of a stint

angiosarcoma [AN-jee-oh-sar-KOH-ma] malignant tumor of blood vessels

angiospasm [AN-jee-oh-spazm] sudden, painful, involuntary contraction of the muscles associated with the blood vessels

angiostenosis [an-jee-oh-steh-NOH-sis] narrowed lumen of a blood vessel

angiotensin I [an-jee-oh-TEN-sin won] a physically inactive hormone that is a converted into angiotensin II by the lungs

angiotensin II [an-jee-oh-TEN-sin too] a hormone that increases blood pressure and stimulates production and secretion of aldosterone

anhedonia [AN-hee-DOH-nee-ah] inability to experience pleasure from any activity

anicteric [AN-ik-TER-ik] appearance of being without jaundice

anions [AN-eye-onz] ions with a negative charge

anisocoria [an-EYE-soh-KO-ree-ah] unequal sizes of the pupils, often caused by glaucoma, head trauma, stroke, or a tumor that causes the iris to dilate and constrict

anisocytosis [an-EYE-soh-sy-TOH-sis] an increase in variation of the size of cells, frequently used in reference to red blood cells

ankylosing spondylitis [ang-kih-LOH-sing SPAWN-dih-LYE-tis] chronic inflammation of the vertebrae that leads to fibrosis, restricted movement of the vertebrae, and stiffening of the spine; treatment includes nonsteroidal anti-inflammatory agents

annulus fibrosis [AN-yoo-lus figh-BRO-sus] layer of fibrocartilage surrounding each intervertebral disc

anorexia [an-oh-REK-see-ah] loss of appetite

anorexia nervosa [an-oh-REK-see-ah nur-VOH-suh] disorder characterized by not eating due to a morbid fear of weight gain, resulting in severe emaciation

anosmia [an-OZ-mee-ah] loss of the sense of smell

ant- [ant] *prefix*; apart or excessive

antacids [ant-AS-idz] agents used to neutralize acids, most commonly in the stomach

ante- [an-tee] *prefix*; before

ante cibum (a.c.) [AHN-tee cee-BUM] abbreviated a.c. when written in medical instructions or physician orders, this indicates that medication or treatment is administered before meals

anteflexion [an-tee-FLECK-shun] bending forward a part of an organ; normal position of the uterus as it bends forward over the bladder

anterior [an-TEER-ee-or] front of the body

anterior chamber of the eye [an-TEER-ee-or CHAM-ber uv the eye] area immediately behind the cornea and in front of the lens of the eye

anterior cruciate ligament [an-TEER-ee-or KROO-shee-ayt LIG-ah-ment] a band of strong fibrous tissue originating on the front of the femur and inserting on the tibia, acting to stabilize the knee; injuries to this area of the knee are common in athletes

anterior tibial muscle [an-TEER-ee-or TIB-ee-al MUS-sel] muscle of front surface of the lower leg that flexes and abducts the foot when contracted

anterior tibial vein [an-TEER-ee-or TIB-ee-al vayn] blood vessel that returns blood to the femoral vein from the lower leg

anterograde amnesia [AN-ter-oh-grayd am-NEE-zee-ah] lack of ability to recall events after a specific event such as a trauma or administration of a medication

anteroposterior [AN-ter-oh-pohs-TEER-ee-or] from the front to the back of the body

anteversion [an-tee-VER-shun] forward tilting of organ or part of an organ; forward tilting of uterus over the bladder

anthracosis [an-thruh-KOH-sis] lung disease caused by inhalation of coal dust; also known as "black lung disease"

anthropometric measurements [an-thro-po-MET-trik MEH-zur-mentz] measurement of the size, weight, and proportions of the body

anti- [an-tee] *prefix*; opposed or against

antianaphylaxis [an-tee-an-ah-fi-LAK-sis] a procedure for making a person insensitive to an antigen; desensitization

antiarrhythmic drug [an-tee-ah-RITH-mik drug] pharmacological agents that control or prevent irregular or abnormal heart rhythms

antibiotics [AN-tee-by-AWT-ik] category of medications that treat bacterial infections

antibody [AN-tih-bod-ee] proteins produced by plasma cells in response to foreign substances such as bacteria, viruses, and toxins

anticholinergic [AN-tee-kol-ih-NER-Jik] a class of medications that antagonize actions of the parasympathetic and other cholinergic nerve fibers

anticoagulants [an-tee-ko-AG-yoo-lants] class of medications that delay or prevent clot formation

anticonvulsants [AN-tee-kon-VUL-santz] pharmacological agents that raise the seizure threshold or prevent seizure activity

antidepressant [AN-tee-dee-PRES-ant] medications used to improve mood and resolve depression; classes include bicyclic, tetracyclic, and monoamine oxidase (MAO) inhibitors

antidiabetic drug [AN-tee-dy-ah-BET-ik drug] medications that act to stabilize blood glucose metabolism by stimulation of insulin or replacement

antidote [AN-tee-doht] a specific agent that works to counteract a poison or its effect

antiemetic [AN-tee-eh-MET-ik] category of medications used to treat nausea, vomiting, and motion sickness

antiflatulants [an-tee-FLAT-yoo-lantz] pharmacological agents that diminish the formation of gases in the colon

antigens [AN-tee-jenz] substances, usually proteins, that cause the formation of antibodies and react specifically with that antibody

antihistamines [an-tee-HIS-tah-meenz] pharmacological agents used to counteract histamine; frequently used for allergic response

anti-inflammatory [AN-tee-in-FLAM-ah-toh-ree] pharmacological agents used to reduce the bodily responses without affecting the cause of inflammation

antineoplastics [AN-tee-nee-oh-PLAS-tiks] pharmacological agents that prevent the development and spread of neoplastic cells

antinuclear antibodies (ANA) [an-tee-NYOO-klee-ar AN-tih-bod-eez] immunoglobulin produced by the body that acts against its own nuclear material, indicative of autoimmune diseases such as systemic lupus erythematosus and rheumatoid arthritis

antinuclear antibody test [an-tee-NYOO-klee-ar AN-tih-bod-ee test] blood test used in the diagnosis of autoimmune diseases

antioxidants [an-tee-OX-sih-dants] substances that block or inhibit destructive oxidation reactions

antipruritics [an-tee-pru-RIT-iks] pharmacological agents that prevent or reduce itching

antipsychotic [an-tee-sigh-KAW-tik] pharmacological agents used to treat psychosis, paranoia, and schizophrenia by blocking dopamine receptors in the limbic system; also known as neuroleptics and major tranquilizers; classes include phenothiazines, high-potency agents, typical and atypical antipsychotics

antipyretics [AN-tee-pye-RET-iks] pharmacological agents such as aspirin and acetaminophen that reduce fever

antisepsis [an-tee-SEP-sis] measures taken to prevent exposure and growth of infectious agents

antisocial personality [AN-tee-SOH-shal per-son-AL-ih-tee] a psychiatric disorder characterized by disregard of rules, laws, morals, and ethics of society; demonstrated by lying, stealing, manipulation, and the inability to feel remorse for exploiting others

antispasmodic [AN-tee-spaz-MOD-ik] pharmacological agent that reduces or eliminates cramping or irregular and painful involuntary muscular contractions

antitoxin [AN-tee-tok-sin] serum antibody formed in response to a biological toxin that works to counteract a specific poisonous substance

antitussives [an-tee-TUS-ivz] pharmacological agents that suppress cough

antrum [AHN-trum] section of the stomach that terminates at the pylorus

anuria [an-YOO-ree-ah] absence of urine output or a quantity of 100 mL daily

anus [AYE-nus] circular, external opening of the rectum, controlled by the anal sphincter

anxiolytic [ANG-zee-oh-LIT-ik] pharmacological classification of drugs that relieve anxiety and stress

aorta [aye-OR-tah] largest artery, arises from the left ventricle

aortalgia [aye-or-TAL-jee-ah] pain caused by an aneurysm or other disorders of the aorta

aortic coarctation [aye-OR-tik ko-ark-TAY-shun] congenital narrowing of the aorta

aortic stenosis [aye-OR-tik ste-NOH-sis] obstruction or narrowing of the aortic valve causing significant reduction of blood flow from the left ventricle, resulting in decreased cardiac output

aortic valve [aye-OR-tik valv] valve located between the left ventricle and the ascending aorta

aortoplasty [ay-or-toh-PLAS-tee] surgical repair of the aorta

ap- [ap] *prefix*; separated or derived from

apathy [AP-ah-thee] lacking interest, indifference associated with major depression and other psychiatric conditions

aperture [AP-er-chur] entrance to a body cavity or channel

apex [AYE-pex] end point of an organ or structure

aphagia [ah-FAY-jee-ah] inability to swallow

aphakia [ah-FAY-kee-ah] condition in which the lens of the eye has been surgically removed or is absent

aphalangia [ah-fah-LAN-jee-ah] lacking fingers or toes

aphasia [ah-FAY-see-ah] condition without speech; may be defined further as expressive or receptive types

apheresis [aye-FER-ee-sis] a therapeutic procedure that separates out one specific type of blood cell, then reinfuses the remaining blood to the patient as a trans-fusion to remove harmful elements from the blood

aphonia [aye-FOH-nee-ah] loss of speaking voice, usually due to irritation, infection, and swelling of the larynx

aphthous stomatitis [AF-thus sto-mah-TYE-tis] canker sores, present as small ulcers of the oral mucosa

apical [AYE-pi-kul] heartbeat heard at the apex of the heart

aplastic anemia [aye-PLAS-tik ah-NEE-mee-ah] deficiency of blood cells resulting from failure of the bone marrow to produce adequate numbers of circulating blood cells; may be congenital or acquired

apnea [AP-nee-uh] cessation of respiration

apneustic area [ap-NEW-stik AIR-ee-uh] the brain region responsible for coordination of movements and activities essential for transition from inspiration and exhalation

apo- [aye-poh] *prefix*; away from

aponeurosis [AP-oh-nu-ROH-sis] fibrous tendon sheets that serve as attachments for muscular fibers and sometimes function as a fascia for muscles; plural is aponeuroses

aponeurotic fibroma [aye-poh-new-ROH-tik figh-BROH-mah] a recurrent nonmetastasizing infiltrating calcification observed most often on the palms of young patients as a small, firm nodule not attached to the dermal layer

apoplexia [ap-oh-PLEK-see-uh] sudden, gross bleeding in an organ; stroke caused by bleeding in the brain

appendectomy [ap-pen-DEK-toh-mee] surgical removal of the appendix due to infection and/or rupture

appendiceal [AP-en-DIH-see-al] pertaining to appendix

appendicitis [ah-PEN-dih-SY-tis] inflammation of the appendix with severe pain

appendicular skeleton [ap-PEN-dik-yoo-lar SKEL-eh-ton] the bones of the limbs and girdles attached to the axial skeleton

appendix [ah-PEN-diks] a thin, tubular, closed-ended section of the bowel located off the cecum that has no role in the digestive process

apperception [AP-per-SEP-shun] the process of clearly perceiving one's own personality

apraxia [aye-PRAKS-ee-ah] inability to use or manipulate objects while still being able to name and describe how the object is used

aqueous humor [ah-kwee-us HYOO-mor] a clear, watery fluid that is continuously probated by the ciliary processes in the posterior chamber of the eye

-ar [ahr] *suffix*; pertaining to

arachnoid layer [ah-RAK-noyd LAY-er] the middle layer of the three meninges covering the central nervous system

arbor vitae [AHR-bur VYE-tay] a treelike structural outline seen in the cerebellum which is visible on computerized tomography scans and other imaging studies

-arche [ark-ee] *suffix*; beginning or start

areflexia [ah-re-FLEK-see-ah] lack of reflex or response to verbal, sensory, or pain stimulation

-arian [ar-ee-an] *suffix*; pertaining to a person

-aris [ar-is] *suffix*; pertaining to

arousal [ah-ROWZ-ahl] component linked closely to the appearance of wakefulness and alertness

arrector pili [ah-REK-tor PYE-lye] muscles attached to hair follicles that cause "goose bumps" when involuntarily contracted

arrhythmia [ah-RITH-mee-ah] loss of regular rate or rhythm of heartbeat

arterial blood gases [ar-TEE-ree-al BLUD gas-ez] a laboratory study measuring the oxygen and carbon dioxide in a sample obtained from an arterial blood sample

arterioles [ar-TEER-ee-olz] smallest branches of arteries

arteriopathy [ar-TEE-ree-OP-ah-thee] collective term for disease of artery

arteriorrhaphy [ar-tee-ree-OR-ah-fee] suturing of an artery

arteriorrhexis [ar-tee-ree-oh-REK-sis] rupture of an artery

arteriosclerosis [ar-teer-ee-oh-skle-ROH-sis] hardening of the arteries

arteriosclerosis obliterans [ar-teer-ee-oh-skle-ROH-sis oh-BLIT-er-anz] a gradual narrowing of the arteries with thrombosis and degeneration of the intima

arteriostenosis [ar-tee-ree-oh-steh-NO-sis] narrowing of an artery

arteriovenous fistula [ar-teer-ee-oh-VEE-nus FIST-yoo-luh] a surgical joining of arterial and venous vessels in order to gain access to circulation during hemodialysis

artery [AR-tur-ee] vessel carrying blood away from the heart

arthralgia [ar-THRAL-gee-ah] pain in the joint from injury, inflammation, or infection

arthrocentesis [ar-throh-sen-TEE-sis] removal of excess fluid in a joint by inserting a needle into the joint space

arthrodesis [AR-throh-DEE-sis] surgical procedure to fuse the bones in a degenerate or unstable joint

arthrogram [AR-throh-gram] MRI, x-ray, or CT images of a joint and adjoining structures

arthrography [ar-THROG-ra-fee] a radiological procedure that uses a radiopaque injection into a joint that coats and outlines the bone ends and joint capsule

arthropathy [ar-THRO-path-ee] any disease of a joint, including inflammatory and hereditary disorders

arthroplasty [AR-thro-PLAS-tee] surgical replacement of a joint; often required due to degenerative joint changes

arthroscopy [ar-THROS-koh-pee] surgical procedure that uses a fiberoptic scope to visualize a joint and remove tissues such as damaged cartilage or bone spurs

articular cartilage [ar-TIK-yoo-lar KAR-tih-lij] the smooth, nonvascular, dense connective tissue that covers the end surfaces of bones forming synovial joints

-ary [air-ee] *suffix*; pertaining to

asaphia [ah-SAF-ee-ah] inability to produce clear and distinct speech

asbestosis [as-bes-TOH-sis] pneumoconiosis caused by inhalation of asbestosis fibers, usually from occupational exposure

ascending colon [ah-SEN-ding KOH-lon] segment of the bowel that extends upward on the right side of the abdomen, joining the transverse colon

ascites [ah-SY-teez] accumulation of excess fluid in the peritoneal cavity; most commonly caused by cirrhosis of the liver due to alcoholism, but also from heart failure and kidney disease

-ase [ace] or [ays] *suffix*; enzyme

aseptic [aye-SEP-tik] free from infectious material

aspartate aminotransferase test (AST) [as-PAR-tate ah-meen oh TRANS-fer-ace test] intracellular enzyme test to detect tissue damage in the liver, brain, and muscles

Asperger's disorder [AS-per-gers dis-OR-der] a developmental disorder characterized by poor social skills, repetitive behaviors, and focused interest in an esoteric topic that limits social and occupational functioning

asphyxia [as-FIK-see-ah] suffocation resulting from impaired or absent oxygen exchange

aspiration [as-pi-RAY-shun] removal of fluid or accumulation from the body by suction; inhalation of a substance or object into the airway such as food, drink, or vomitus

aspiration pneumonia [as-pi-RAY-shun noo-MOH-nee-ah] lung infection caused by foreign material entering the lung

assist-control ventilation [ah-SIST kon-TROL ven-tih-LAY-shun] mechanically supported breathing where the patient is permitted to initiate breathing but the ventilator delivers a preset volume of air and will initiate breathing if the patient's breathing slows or stops

astasia [ah-STA-zee-ah] inability to stand or maintain erect posture due to muscular incoordination

asterixis [as-ter-IK-sis] gross, involuntary, jerking tremor of the hand; also called flapping tremor

asterognosis [ah-STEER-ee-og-NOH-sis] inability to discern an object by touch alone

asthenia [as-THEE-nee-ah] lacking strength; weakness; often refers to muscular or cerebellar diseases

-asthenia [as-theen-ee-ah] *suffix*; weakness, decreased strength

asthma [AZ-mah] disease of the respiratory system characterized by increased airway irritability, narrowing and constriction of the air passages

asthmatic [az-MAT-ik] patient with asthma

astrocytoma [as-tro-sy-TOH-mah] malignant tumor of the brain or spinal cord composed of astrocytes, with typical onset in the fifth decade of life

asymmetry [aye-SIM-eh-tree] clinical finding of dissimilar proportion in two normally similar body parts

asymptomatic [AYE-simp-toh-MAT-ik] not demonstrating external signs or complaints of a disease

asynchronous pacing [aye-syn-KRON-us PAYS-ing] electrical stimulation of the heart that sets a rate that is independent of the heart's own pacemakers

asynclitism [ah-SIN-kli-tizm] presentation of the fetal head in an oblique position during labor

asyndesis [ah-SIN-de-sis] a brain disorder characterized by the inability to bring thoughts together to form a cohesive concept

asyntaxia [ah-sin-TAK-see-ah] lack of appropriate and orderly development of an embryo

asystole [aye-SIS-toe-lee] lack of heartbeat; cardiac standstill

atasia [ah-TAYZ-ee-ah] inability of the muscles of the digestive tract to relax

ataxia [aye-TAK-see-ah] uncoordinated muscle activity; spastic or jerky motions

-ate [ayte] *suffix*; pertaining to or composed of

atelectasis [AT-eh-LEK-tah-sis] collapse of lung tissue resulting in impaired gaseous exchange

atherectomy [ath-eh-REK-toh-mee] surgical removal of a fatty or lipid deposit (atheroma) in an artery

atheromatous plaque [ath-er-OH-may-tus PLAK] an area of swelling in the lining of an artery due to deposits of lipids

atherosclerosis [ATH-er-oh-skle-ROH-sis] plaque formation on the inner arterial wall of a blood vessel

atherosclerotic plaque [ATH-er-oh-skle-roh-tik plak] thick, hard deposit on the walls of the inner arteries that can clog the arteries in the heart and the brain or other organs

athetosis [ath-eh-TOH-sis] involuntary, slow, and irregular snakelike, twisting movements in the upper extremities associated with encephalitis, cerebral palsy, hepatic encephalopathy, Huntington's chorea, or drug toxicity

-ation [aye-shun] *suffix*; process of having or being

-ative [ah-tiv] *suffix*; pertaining to

atlas [AT-las] the first cervical vertebra (C1) located directly below the occipital bone of the cranium

atonic bladder [aye-TON-ik BLAD-er] inability to completely empty the urinary bladder; often associated with paralysis and diabetic neuropathy

atony [aye-TON-ee] lacking normal tension; flaccid or relaxed

atopic dermatitis [ay-TOP-ick dur-muh-TYE-tis] skin inflammation of genetic origin

atopognosis [ah-top-og-NOH-sis] inability to correctly identify the location of a tactile sensation

atopy [AT-uh-pee] a genetically determined allergic or hypersensitive response

atresia [ah-TREE-zee-ah] absence of a normal orifice, duct, or canal such as the auditory or biliary canals

atreto- [ah-tret-oh] *prefix*; lack of a normally occurring opening

atrial ectopic beats (AEB) [AYE-tree-al ek-TOP-ik beets] early or out-of-sequence contraction of the atrium of the heart

atrial fibrillation [AYE-tree-al fib-ril-LAY-shun] rapid, irregular twitching of the upper chambers of the heart

atrial septal defect [AYE-tree-al SEP-tul DEE-fekt] an abnormal opening between the atria permitting blood to shunt back and forth

atrioseptoplasty [aye-tree-oh-SEP-toh-plas-tee] surgical repair of a defect in the partition between the atria of the heart

atrioventricular canal (AV canal) [AYE-tree-oh-ven-TRIK-yoo-lar ka-NAL] refers to a combination of defects in the atrial and ventricular septa and portions of tricuspid and mitral valves

atrioventricular node (AV node) [AYE-tree-oh-ven-TRIK-yoo-lar nohd] an area of specialized cardiac muscle that receives electrical impulses from the sinoatrial node and sends impulses to the ventricles, causing them to contract

atrioventricular valve [AYE-tree-oh-ven-TRIK-yoo-lar valv] the bicuspid (mitral) and tricuspid valves located between the atria and ventricles

atrium [AYE-tree-uhm] two upper heart chambers directly above the ventricles, called right and left atrium, respectively

atrophy [AT-roh-fee] muscle tissue wasting as a result of disuse, ischemia, or nutritional deficiencies

attending behaviors [at-TEND-ing BEE-hav-yehrs] nonverbal signs indicating focused listening, or interest in what another person is communicating

attention-deficit hyperactivity disorder (ADHD) [ah-TEN-shun DEF-eh-sit HIGH-per-ak-TIV-it-ee dis-OR-der] distractibility, short attention span, inability to follow directions, restlessness, hyperactivity, labile mood, and impulsiveness; may be caused by mild brain damage at birth, genetic factors, or other abnormalities

attenuated vaccine [ah-TEN-yoo-aye-ted vak-SEEN] vaccine in which the antigen's ability to produce disease has been lessened or eliminated by heat or chemical measures; after inoculation, mild symptoms may result

-ature [ah-tur] suffix; system composed of

audiometry [aw dee OM-eh-tree] process of measuring a patient's hearing ability

auditory [AW-dih-tor-ee] pertaining to hearing processes

auditory aphasia [AW-dih-tor-ee ah-FAY-zee-ah] impaired comprehension of spoken words in the presence of normal hearing

auditory aura [AW-dih-tor-ee AW-rah] abnormal sensations of sound that precede a seizure

auditory canal [AW-dih-tor-ee ka-NAL] opening of the external ear that leads from the external auditory meatus to the tympanic membrane

auditory channel [AW-dih-tor-ee CHAN-nul] transmission of messages through spoken words and cues

auditory nerve [AW dih-tor-ee NERV] eighth cranial nerve; conducts impulses from the semicircular canals and the cochlea to the brain to maintain balance and the sense of hearing

auditory ossicles [AW-di-tor-ee OS-ih-kulz] small bones of the ear: malleus, incus, and stapes

augmented cough [awg-MEN-ted kawf] method of increasing force and effectiveness of chest muscles by placing the palm of the hand on the abdominal musculature below the ribs during expiration and then removing the hand during inspiration

aural [AW-ral] pertaining to the ear

auricle [AW-ri-kul] tissue and cartilage that form the C shape of the external ear and semicircular canals

auris dexter [AW-ris DEKS-ter] right ear

auris sinistra [AW-ris SIN-is-trah] left ear

auscultation [AWS-kul-TAY-shun] use of a stethoscope to listen to heart, lungs, and bowel sounds

auscultatory gap [AWS-kul-tay-tor-ee GAP] temporary disappearance of sounds at the end of Korotkoff phase I and the beginning of phase II while listening with a stethoscope

autism [AW-tizm] neuropsychological condition characterized by limited social and communication abilities and rigidly adhering to routines and internal thoughts

auto- [AW-toh] *prefix;* self

autoimmune disorders [aw-toh-i-MEWN dis-OR-ders] conditions in which the immune response is directed toward the self

autologous transfusion [aw-TOL-oh-gus trans-FYOO-shun] infusion of a previously donated unit of a patient's own blood to correct loss during surgery or other interventions

automaticity [aw-toh-mah-TISS-uh-tee] ability to contract without neural stimulation

autopsy [AW-top-see] postmortem examination to determine the cause of death

autoregulation [AW-toe-reg-yoo-LAY-shun] redistribution of blood flow to areas of greatest need; self-management of emotions and behavior during periods of stress

autosomal chromosomes [aw-toh-SOW-mal KRO-moh-sohmz] the 22 pairs of chromosomes that are responsible for characteristics other than determination of sex

avascular [ah-VAS-kyoo-lar] characteristic of few or no blood vessels

aversion therapy [ah-VUHR-shun THER-ah-pee] use of an unpleasant sensation or association to decrease destructive behaviors such as drug and alcohol abuse; noxious stimuli may range from mild electrical shock or smells like ammonia

axilla [AK-sil-ah] region below the junction of the shoulder joint; armpit

axillary lymph nodes [AK-si-lar-ee limf nodz] lymphatic structures that collect chyme in the area below the shoulder and armpit

axis [AX-iss] the second cervical vertebrae (C2)

axon [AK-son] structural process of a nerve cell that conducts nervous impulses away from the cell body and dendrites

AY4 antibodies [AYE-why-for AN-tih-bod-eez] substances produced in the body that react to an antigen

azotemia [az-oh-tee-mee-ah] abnormal concentration of urea and nitrogenous substances in the blood caused by failure of the kidneys

B

B lymphocyte [bee LIM-foh-syt] cells that are produced in the bone marrow that travel to the lymph nodes and other lymphoid tissue, becoming part of the body's immune system by producing antibodies

Babinski sign [bah-BIN-skee sine] extension of the great toe and abduction of the other toes when the plantar surface of the foot is stimulated; indicative of pyramidal tract involvement

bacterial vaginosis [bak-TEE-reh-al vaj-ih-NOH-sis] a condition caused by a disruption of normal bacterial flora in the vagina causing irritation to and drainage from the vagina

bacteriuria [bak-teer-ee-YOO-ree-ah] presence of bacteria in the urine; when bacterial count rises above 100,000 per mL of urine, it indicates a urinary tract infection

bag-valve mask [bag-valv mask] a manually operated resuscitation device used to ventilate a nonbreathing patient; the device consists of a reservoir bag, a unidirectional valve, and a face mask

Baker's cyst [BAY-kerz sist] a collection of fluid in the synovium of the popliteal fossa behind the knee

balanitis [bal-ah-NY-tis] inflammation of the skin covering the glans penis which may result from sexually transmitted diseases

Banti's syndrome [BAN-teez SIN-drom] condition characterized by anemia, enlarged spleen and hemorrhages, culminating in cirrhosis of the liver due to portal hypertension

baragnosis [bar-ag-NOH-sis] inability to estimate weight of objects, indicates presence of a parietal lobe lesion

bariatrics [bar-ee-AT-riks] a branch of medicine focused on treatment and management of obesity

barium enema [BAIR-ee-yum EN-eh-ma] infusion of radiopaque barium into the lower intestinal tract for fluoroscopic study

barium swallow [BAIR-ee-yum SWAL-oh] radiographic study of the phalanx and esophagus after ingestion of barium sulfate

baroreceptor [BAR-oh-ree-SEP-tor] nerve endings in the cardiovascular system that regulate blood pressure by responding to relative pressure within

barotitis media [bar-oh-TYE-tis MEE-dee-uh] middle ear inflammation caused by changes in atmospheric pressure, such as in a descending airplane or in deep-sea diving

barotrauma [bar-oh-TRAW-mah] damage to alveoli resulting from mechanical ventilation

barrel chest [BARE-el chest] an increase in the anteroposterior diameter of the chest such that it resembles a barrel rather than a normal oval shape

Barret esophagus [BAR-et ee-SOF-ah-gus] long-standing irritation and ulceration of the distal esophagus associated with increased risk for adenocarcinoma

Barthel Self-Care Index [BAHR-tel self-kare IN-deks] standardized screening tool used in older adults for measuring ability to perform self-care

basal cell carcinoma [BAY-sal sel kahr-si-NOH-muh] malignancy of the basal cell layer

basal metabolic rate (BMR) [BAY-sal met-ah-BOL-ik rayt] physiological consumption of calories as measured 12 hours after eating, sleeping, and being at complete rest

basement membrane [DAYS-ment MEM-brayn] a delicate noncellular layer of pliable tissue that serves as support and attachment for epithelial cells

basophil [BAY-soh-fil] one type of white blood cell comprising less than 1 percent of all leukocytes

Behçet's syndrome [BAY-sets SIN-drom] a multisystemic chronic and recurrent disease characterized by oral and genital ulcerations and uveitis of the eyes resulting in blindness

Bell's palsy [BELLZ PAWL-zee] temporary, peripheral, unilateral paralysis of the muscles innervated by the facial nerve that causes distorted facial expressions, ptosis, tearing, and salivation on the affected side

belonephobia [BEL-oh-nee-FOH-bee-ah] morbid fear of needles and other objects with sharp points

Bence-Jones protein [bents-jonz PRO-teenz] a protein found in urine of individuals with multiple myeloma

Benedikt's syndrome [BEN-eh-dikts SIN-drom] paralysis of one side of the body with spasms or tremors, and occulomotor paralysis on the opposite side

benign [bee-NINE] not malignant, condition of mild intensity

benign familial polyposis [bee-NINE fah-MIL-ee-al POL-ee-POH-sis] a hereditary condition characterized by multiple benign colonic polyps which can become malignant

benign prostatic hypertrophy [be-NINE proh-STAT-ik high-PER-troh-fee] enlargement of the prostate gland associated with age that is not malignant but may present obstruction of urine flow

beryllosis [be-ril-ee-OH-sis] pneumoconiosis caused by inhalation of beryllium salts

beta adrenergic blocking agents [BAY-tah ad-reh-NER-jik BLOK-ing AYE-jentz] pharmacological class of agents that occupy beta receptor sites

beta waves [BAY-tah wayvz] brain activity that is typical of increased neural activity

biceps brachii [BY-seps BRAY-kee-eye] the two muscles of the upper arm that flex the forearm and flex the hand when contracted

biceps femoris [BY-seps fem-OR-is] one of the posterior lateral muscles of the thigh included in the hamstring group that causes external rotation and flexion of the hip when contracted

bicuspid [bi-KUS-pid] having two points or parts

bicuspid valve [bye-KUS-pid valv] valve between the left atrium and the left ventricle; left atrioventricular valve, mitral valve

bifurcation [bi-fer-KAY-shun] to divide into two branches

bigeminy [bi-JEM-ih-nee] paired occurrences, such as heart rhythms

bilateral [bi-LAT-er-al] pertaining to having two sides

bile [BIHL] the fluid produced by the liver, stored in the gallbladder, released into the duodenum to digest fats in foods

bile duct [BIHL dukt] the tubular structure that bile flows through

biliary [BIL-ee-air-ee] pertaining to bile, gall

biliary atresia [BIL-ee-air-ee ah-TREE-zee-ah] congenital absence of major bile ducts; also called neonatal hepatitis

biliary cirrhosis [BIL-ee-air-ee sir-ROH-sis] liver disorder due to obstructed bile ducts

biliary tract [BIL-ee-air-ee trakt] collective term for structures involved in the delivery of bile from the liver to the duodenum; includes the gallbladder, hepatic ducts, cystic ducts, and common bile ducts

bilirubin [BIL-ih-ROO-bin] end product from the breakdown of old red blood cells

bilirubin level [BIL-ih-ROO-bin LEV-el] blood test for unconjugated, conjugated, and total bilirubin levels; levels are abnormal when there is biliary obstruction or liver disease

biliverdin [BIL-ih-VER-din] a greenish bile pigment; gall substance

Billroth's I operation [BIL-rothz wun op-er-AYE-shun] surgical removal of the pylorus and antrum of the stomach with attachment of the stomach to the duodenum; also known as gastroduodenostomy

Billroth's II operation [BIL-rothz too op-er-AYE-shun] surgical removal of the pylorus and antrum with closure of the ends of the stomach and duodenum, followed by attaching the stomach to the jejunum; also known as gastrojejunostomy

bin- [bine] *prefix*; twice or double

bioavailability [by-oh-ah-VAIL-ah-BIL-ih-tee] readiness of a drug to produce an effect in the circulation at the target site

biopsy [BY-op-see] a surgical procedure to obtain a tissue sample of a mass, tumor, or skin lesion for the purpose of cellular study

biot respirations [bee-OH res-pi-RAY-shunz] periods of apnea alternating with breaths of the same depth

bipolar disorder [by-POH-lar dis-OR-der] a mood disorder characterized by abnormally high and low moods and severe behavioral disturbance

bladder [BLAD-der] a saclike structure that acts as a receptacle for secretions; term generally refers to the urinary bladder

bladder neck suspension [BLAD-der NEK sus-PEN-shun] surgical fixation of the urethrovesical junction and the bladder neck to an elevated retropubic position to alleviate stress incontinence

-blast [blast] *suffix*; immature cell

blepharitis [BLEF-ah-RY-tis] inflammation or infection of the eyelid with redness, exudate, and scales at the bases of the eyelashes

blepharoplasty [BLEF-ah-roh-plas-tee] surgical revision of the eyelid

blepharoptosis [BLEF-ah-rop-TOH-sis] drooping of the upper eyelid tissue due to diseases that affect the muscles or nerves of the eye, such as myasthenia gravis or stroke

blepharospasm [BLEF-ah-roh-spazm] involuntary contraction of muscles of the eyelid

blind spot [BLYND spot] portion of the retina that has no ability to perceive images

blood pressure [BLUD presh-ur] force exerted by the circulating blood on the arterial walls at the points of contraction (diastolic) and filling (systolic)

blood urea nitrogen [BLUD YOO-ree-uh NIH-troh-jen] a diagnostic blood test; determines the amount of urea present in the blood that is directly related to the metabolic function of the liver and excretory function of the kidney

blood-brain barrier [blud-brain BAR-ee-er] selective mechanism that prevents passage of toxic or large chemicals into the brain while permitting essential substances such as oxygen and glucose to enter

B-lymphocytes [bee-LIM-foh-sightz] cells that produce antibodies that travel through the blood with the ability to attach to foreign cells, labeling them for destruction by phagocytes

-body [boh-dee] *suffix*; thing or structure

body alignment [BOH-dee ah-LYNE-ment] position of body parts in relation to each other or with regard to normal posture

body dysmorphic disorder [BOH-dee dis-MOR-fik dis-OR der] preoccupation with minor defects in the appearance of the body, particularly the face, with the demand for frequent plastic surgery

-bol [bol] *suffix*; throw

bolus [BOH-lus] a mass of chewed food or medicine that is ready to be swallowed

bonding [BON-ding] formation of attachment between parent and child; adhesion of one substance to another

bone autograft [BOWN AW-toh-graft] procedure of using bone taken from the patient's own body to use to stabilize and fuse with bony structures

bone densitometry [BOWN DEN-sih-TAWM-eh-tree] refers to two types of bone density tests: dual-energy x-ray absorptiometry (DEXA) scan, and quantitative computerized topography (QCT) which determines the degree of bone mineralization

bone marrow [BOWN mar-row] tissue in the central cavity of long bones that functions to store fat or produce red blood cells

bone marrow aspiration [BOWN mar-row as-pih-RAY-shun] procedure to remove red bone marrow from the posterior iliac crest of the hipbone

bony labyrinth [BOWN-ee LAB-ih-rinth] a series of osseous chambers located within the temporal bone; essential to hearing

borderline personality [BOR-der-lyne per-soh-NAL-it-ee] a psychiatric disorder characterized by an inability to sustain stable relationships, fear of abandonment, hypersensitivity, changeable emotions, poor tolerance to stress, and overdependence

botulism [BOT-yoo-liz-um] illness acquired by ingesting improperly cooked or canned food containing *Clostridium botulinum*; causes paralysis and is potentially fatal

Bowman's capsule [BOW-manz KAP-sool] a cup-shaped structure that encloses the glomerulus in the renal tubule or nephron; also known as the glomerular capsule

brachial artery [BRAY-kee-ul AR-tur-ee] main blood vessel bringing blood to the arm, branching off the subclavian artery and terminating at the cubital fossa of the elbow

brachial plexus [BRAY-kee-ul PLEK-sus] spinal nerve network of the lower cervical and first thoracic nerves

brachial veins [BRAY-kee-ul vaynz] main blood vessel that returns blood from the arm, terminating at the axillary vein

brachialis muscle [bray-kee-AY-lis MUS-sel] muscle that flexes the forearm

brachiocephalic [BRAY-kee-oh-seh-FAL-ik] pertaining to the arm and head

brachiocephalic lymph duct [BRAY-kee-oh-seh-FAL-ik limf dukt] vessel that drains chyme from the arm

brachiocephalic vein [BRAY-kee-oh-seh-FAL-ik vayn] major blood vessel formed by the union of the internal jugular and subclavian veins that returns blood from the head and neck region

brachiocyllosis [BRAY-kee-oh-sil-OH-sis] an abnormal curvature of the arm

brachioradialis muscle [BRAY-kee-oh-ray-dee-AL-is MUS-sel] muscle of the lateral forearm that flexes the wrist when contracted; attached at the head of the radius

-brachy [bray-key] *suffix*; short

brady- [bray-dee] *prefix*; slow, decreased rate

bradycardia [bray-dee-KAR-dee-ah] abnormally slowed heart rate; less than 60 beats per minute in an adult

bradyglossia [bray-dee-GLOSS-ee-ah] very slow or difficult tongue movement

bradykinesia [bray-dee-kih-NEE-see-uh] abnormally slow movement

bradyphrasia [bray-dee-FRAY-zee-uh] abnormally slow speech

bradyphrenia [bray-dee-FREN-ee-uh] slowed thinking associated with dementia

bradypnea [brad-ip-NEE-uh] abnormally slow respiratory rate

Branham's sign [BRAN-hams sighn] compression of an arteriovenous fistula that slows the heart rate

Braxton-Hicks contraction [BRAKS-ton-hiks kon-TRAK-shun] irregular, nonpainful contractions occurring after the first trimester of pregnancy

breech presentation [breech pree-zen-TAY-shun] any position or presentation of the fetus in the pelvis other than head first

brevicollis [brev-ih-KOL-is] having an abnormally short neck

bronchi [BRONK-eye] airway passage branching off the trachea to the right and left lung fields

bronchial asthma [BRONK-ee-ul AZ-mah] form of airway constriction and irritability characterized by episodic dyspnea and bronchial spasm

bronchial tree [BRONK-ee-al tree] an anatomic complex of the trachea and bronchi

bronchiectasis [BRONG-kee-ek-TAY-sis] dilatation of the bronchioles due to chronic inflammatory lung disease

bronchiectosis [brong-kee-ek-TOH-sis] abnormal widening or dilatation of the bronchi or bronchioles as a result of inflammatory disease or obstruction

bronchioles [BRONG-kee-ohlz] the smaller divisions of the bronchial tree that terminate at the alveoli in the lungs

bronchitis [brong-KIGH-tis] an acute or chronic inflammation of the bronchial tubes

bronchodilator [brong-koh-dy-LAY-tor] pharmacological agent that relaxes the muscles of the bronchus, alleviating bronchospasm and increasing airflow into the lungs; used as a symptomatic treatment in conditions such as asthma

bronchogenic pneumonia [brong-koh-JEN-ik noo-MOH-nee-ah] acute inflammation of the bronchioles and alveoli that produces congestion

bronchopneumonia [BRONG-koh-noo-MOH-nee-ah] infection of the airway including the bronchi, bronchioles, and lung tissue

bronchoscope [BRONG-koh-skope] a small-diameter fiberoptic instrument used to visualize and biopsy the upper airway and lung tissue

bronchospasm [BRONG-koh-spaz-um] an involuntary, rapid contraction of the bronchiole smooth muscle

bronchus [BRONG-kus] section of the airway immediately posterior to the main trunk of the trachea that bifurcates into the right and left segments

Brudzinski sign [bryoo-JIN-skee sighn] physical finding associated with meningitis where passive flexion of the neck produces involuntary flexion of the knees and hips

bruise [BRUZE] bleeding into tissue

bruit [BROO-ee] soft blowing sound heard on auscultation, caused by turbulent blood flow

bruxism [BRUKS-izm] teeth-clenching or -grinding, usually occurring during sleep

bubo [BYOO-boh] extremely enlarged, tender lymph node of the groin that may be associated with syphilis, chancroid, or lymphogranuloma venarum

bucca [BUK-ah] cheek; plural is buccae

buccal [BUK-ahl] pertaining to the inside of the cheek

buccal mucosa [BUK-ahl myoo-KOS-ah] innermost surface of the facial cheek

buccinator muscle [BUK-si-nay-tur MUS-sel] ringlike muscle around the mouth used in smiling, compression of the cheeks, and chewing food

bulbourethral glands [BUL-boh-yoo-RE-thral glanz] two small, bulblike glands located on either side of the urethra just below the prostate gland that secrete a fluid component

bulimia [BUH-lim-ee-ah] disorder characterized by episodes of self-induced purging after binging

bullae [BULL-uh; BULL-ee] blister(s), or plebe(s)

bundle branches [BUN-del branch-ez] major conductive pathways of the heart involved in coordination of the heart muscle

bunion [BUN-yun] disorder of the foot associated with swelling and inflammation of the great toe; commonly seen in women who wear narrow-toed shoes

bunionectomy [BUN-yun-EK-toh-mee] surgical procedure to remove the prominent part of a metatarsal bone that is causing the bunion

bursa [BER-sah] a slender, elongated pocket of synovial membrane that contains synovial fluid and acts as a cushion to reduce friction in areas where a tendon rubs against a bone; plural is bursae

bursectomy [bur-SEK-toh-mee] excision of a synovial membrane containing synovial fluid located in areas where tendons pass over bones

bursitis [bur-SY-tis] inflammation of a fluid-filled synovial sac located over a bony prominence or point of articulation between tendon and bone

C

calcaneus [kal-KAY-nee-us] the largest bone of the foot; commonly referred to as the heel

calcitonin [kal-si-TOH-nin] a thyroid hormone that lowers plasma calcium and phosphate ion levels by inhibiting bone resorption; increases renal excretion

calculogenesis [KAL-kyoo-loh-JEN-eh-sis] formation of a stone in an organ or blood vessel

calefacient [KAL-ee-fah-shent] to warm or to make hot, as in applying a hot compress

calix [KAY-liks] a cup-shaped structure within an organ, such as the kidney

Calve-Perthes disease [kal-VAY-PER-tas dis-EEZ] a self-limiting condition occurring in children between the ages of 2 and 12 years in which there is a necrosis of the ossification centers of bone followed by regeneration and recalcification

canal [kah-NAL] a narrow or tubular channel

canal of Schlemm [kah-NAL of shlem] space between the sclera and cornea of the eye that drains aqueous humor from the eye

cancellous tissue [KAN-sel-us TISH-yu] spongy or lattice-like bone formation located in the epiphyses of developing bone

cancer [KAN-ser] malignant, carcinoma

Candida albicans [KAN-dih-dah AL-bih-kanz] a gram-positive yeast organism that causes infections of the mouth, skin, and vagina

candidiasis [KAN-dih-DY-ah-sis] thrush; oral infection caused by the fungus *Candida albicans*, often due to immunosuppression

capillary [KAP-ih-lair-ee] small blood vessel connecting arteries with veins

capitate [KAP-ih-tayt] bone of the hand; used to describe rounded shape of structures

carbuncle [KAHR-bunk-ul] large furuncle

carcinogenic [kar-sih-noh-JEN-ik] substance, agent, or conditions that produce malignant cells

carcinoma [kahr-si-NOH-muh] cancerous cells; tumor or abnormal cells composed of anaplastic or abnormally shaped epithelial cells

carcinoma in situ [kar-si-NOH-mah in SIGH-too] malignant lesion with cellular changes but limited to the immediate tissue; precursor to invasive malignant disease

Cardarelli's sign [kar-da-REL-leez sighn] pulsating, lateral movement of the trachea associated with aortic aneurysm

cardia [KAR-dee-ah] a small area of the stomach at the point nearest the heart where the esophagus joins the stomach

cardiac arrest [KAR-dee-ak ah-REST] sudden stoppage of the heartbeat

cardiac catheterization [KAR-dee-ak kath-e-tur-i-ZAY-shun] a procedure in which a long, flexible tube is inserted into cardiac vessels via a peripheral artery or vein; images produced from the procedure can isolate vessel blockage

cardiac conduction system [KAR-dee-ak kon-DUK-shun SIS-tem] system of impulses guiding heart contraction comprised of the sinoatrial node, atrioventricular node, atrioventricular bundle, right atrium, right and left bundle branches, and Purkinje fibers to produce a heart contraction

cardiac enzyme test [KAR-dee-ak EN-zym test] battery of blood tests performed to determine the presence of cardiac damage by detecting the level of heart muscle enzymes

cardiac notch [KAR-dee-ak notch] anatomical landmark of the lung where the lung tissue indents to allow for the physical presence of the heart

cardiac scan [KAR-dee-ak skan] diagnostic study of the heart using an injection of a radioisotope and subsequent uptake by the myocardium, followed by imagery by a gamma camera of the heart beating; measures the volume of blood pumped by each ventricle

cardiac sphincter [KAR-dee-ak SFINK-ter] a muscular ring in the esophagus that prevents reflux of food from the stomach; also known as the lower esophageal sphincter

cardiac syncope [KAR-dee-ak SIN-koh-pee] transient and sudden loss of consciousness due to inadequate cardiac output associated with bradycardia, tachycardia, or myocardial infarct

cardiac tamponade [KAR-dee-ak tam-puh-NADE] heart compression resulting from accumulation of fluid in the pericardium

cardiac ventricles [KAR-dee-ak VEN-trih-klz] the two lower heart chambers directly below the atrium, called right and left ventricles, respectively

cardioacceleratory center [kar-dee-oh-ak-SEL-ih-rah-tor-ee SEN-ter] sympathetic nerve center that increases the heart rate and strength of contraction

cardioinhibitory center [kar-dee-oh-in-HIB-ih-tor-ee SEN-ter] parasympathetic nervous system area in the brain that monitors the heart rate and strength of contraction

cardiomyopathy [KAR-dee-oh-migh-OP-uh-thee] disease of the heart muscle or myocardium

cardioplegia [KAR-dee-oh-PLAY-jee-ah] deliberate and temporary paralysis of the heart for the purpose of performing surgery on the heart

cardiopulmonary bypass [KAR-dee-oh-PUL-mo-nair-ee BYE-pass] temporary diversion of blood circulation during heart surgery; blood passes through a heart-lung machine that receives deoxygenated blood from the venous side of circulation and then returns oxygenated blood to the patient's arterial side of circulation

cardiorrhexis [KAR-dee-or-reks-is] rupture of the wall of the myocardium

cardiotonic [KAR-dee-oh-TON-ik] exerting a favorable or enhancing effect on the heart, usually increased strength of contractions and cardiac output

cardioversion [KAR-dee-oh-VER-zuhn] use of electrical countershock to restore regular heart rhythm

caries [KAR-eez] areas of destruction of bone or dental enamel

carina [kah-RIH-nah] anatomical structure of a central ridge on a tissue surface

carotid artery [ka-ROT-id AR-ter-ee] the principal blood supply to the head and neck arising off the aortic arch

carotid bruit [ka-ROT-id bru-EE] systolic murmur detectable in the neck but not in the aortic area

carotid endarterectomy [ka-ROT-id end-ar-ter-EK-toh-mee] surgical removal of intra-arterial obstructions such as of the internal carotid artery, reducing the risk for transient ischemic attacks and strokes

carotid pulse [ka-ROT-id puls] systolic pulsation felt at the base of the neck

carotid sinus syndrome [ka-ROT-id SY-nus SIN-drom] condition where stimulation of a hyperactive carotid sinus causes a severe drop in blood pressure due to vasodilation and bradycardia resulting in syncope

carotid transient ischemic attack [ka-ROT-id TRANZ-ee-ent is-KEE-mik ah-TAK] ischemia of the anterior carotid arteries that lasts for 24 hours or less, causing neurological deficits in speech, vision, motor tracts, and balance

carpal [KAR-puhl] pertaining to wrist or carpal bones

carpal bones [KAR-puhl bohnz] osseous structures of the wrist, including the hemad, pisiform, triquetral, lunate, trapezium, trapezoid, capitate, and scaphoid bones

carpal joints [KAR-puhl joynts] articular surfaces of the wrist

carpal tunnel syndrome [KAR-puhl TUN-el SIN-drom] compression of the median nerve of the hand by connective tissue that causes pain, numbness, and loss of strength of the hand

carpoptosis [kar-pop-TOH-sis] damage to the muscles or nerves of the wrist that cause the wrist to be unable to extend

carpus [KAR-pus] wrist

cartilage transplantation [KAR-tih-lij tranz-plan-TAY-shun] surgical procedure that is an alternative to a total knee replacement; used to treat middle-aged adults with degenerative joint disease of the knee to delay the need for total knee replacement surgery

cartilaginous [KAR-tih-LAJ-ih-nus] pertaining to cartilage

caruncle [KAR-ung-kul] a small, fleshy mass

cast [KAST] application of a rigid form around a body part or fracture to stabilize it in a fixed position to facilitate healing

cata- [kat-uh] *prefix*; down

catabolism [ka-TAB-oh-lizm] destructive phase of metabolism

cataplexy [KAT-ah-plek-see] a transient episode of extreme muscular weakness, triggered by extreme emotional states such as fear, anger, or surprise; sudden and uncontrollable urge to sleep associated with narcolepsy

cataracts [KAT-a-rakts] clouding of the lens of the eye; treated by surgical removal and replacement with a prosthetic intraocular lens

catastrophic reaction [kat-ah-STROF-ik ree-AK-shun] disorganized or agitated behavior commonly associated with dementia when the individual faces overwhelming or threatening situations that are beyond his or her coping ability

catatonic schizophrenia [kat-ah-TAWN-ik skitz-oh-FRE-nee-ah] psychiatric disorder characterized by marked disturbance in thought process, stupor, negativism, and rigidity alternating with periods of great excitement

categorical imperative [KAT-ee-gor-ih-kal im-PER-ah-tiv] concept that states that clinicians should act only if the action is based on a principle that is universal

cathartic [ka THAR tic] pharmacological agents that stimulate peristalsis and evacuation of the bowel

catheterization [kath-e-tur-i-ZAY-shun] insertion of a flexible tube into a body cavity for the instillation or withdrawal of fluid

cations [KAT-eye-onz] ions with a positive charge

cauda equina [KAW-dah ee-KWIGH-nah] the bundle of spinal nerves arising from the lumbosacral and lumbar region

cauda equina syndrome [KAW-dah ee-KWIGH nah SIN-drom] compression of nerve roots of the sacral and coccygeal nerves resulting in numbness in the buttocks, genitalia, or thigh along with disturbed bowel and bladder function

caudal [KAW-dal] general directional term pertaining to the tail-end or distal portion of any structure

caudal anesthesia [KAW-dal AN-es-thee-zee-ah] injection of a local analgesic agent into the epidural space of the sacrum

caudal flexure [KAW-dal FLEK-shur] bent section of the lumbosacral region of an embryo

caus- [kaws] *prefix*; burning

causalgia [kaw-SAL-jee-ah] a severe sensation of burning pain, often in an extremity

caut- [kawt] *prefix*; to burn

cauterize [KAW-ter-rize] burning tissue with thermal heat using electricity, steam, laser, or dry ice, often to destroy diseased tissue or coagulate blood vessels

cavitis [kay-VY-tis] inflammation of the vena cava

cavity [KAV-ih-tee] a hollow space in a body organ or structure; in reference to dentition, this term identifies erosion of dental structure

cecocolopexy [see-koh-KOH-low-pek-see] surgical fixation of the cecum

cecum [SEE-kum] a section of bowel located at the first portion of the large intestine that terminates at the appendix

-cele [seel] *suffix*; bulging or hernia

celiac [SEE-lee-ak] pertaining to the abdominal cavity

celiac disease [SEE-lee-ak dis-EEZ] malabsorption disorder caused by gluten sensitivity; celiac sprue

celiac sprue [SEE-lee-ak sproo] gluten enteropathy; a food allergy to the gluten in wheat that causes tissues of the small intestine to become damaged by the allergic response

celiac trunk [SEE-lee-ak trunk] part of the abdominal aorta from which arteries arise to take blood to the stomach, small intestine, liver, gallbladder, and pancreas

cellular infiltration [SEL-you-lar in-fil-TRAY-shun] movement or growth of cells from their usual location by means of unusual growth; often used to describe inflammation and some malignant neoplasms

cellulitis [sell-yoo-LYF-tis] inflammation of connective tissue, especially of the subcutaneous tissue

-centesis [sin-tee-sis] *suffix*; puncture

central fissure [SEN-tral FISH-ur] a central landmark depression on the surface of the liver

central line [SEN-tral lyne] a venous access device inserted into the subclavian vein, used to infuse medications, fluids, and other agents as well as to measure venous pressure

cephalad [SEF-ah-lad] toward or in the direction of the head

cephalalgia [SEF-al-AL-jee-ah] headache

cephalic duct [seh-FAL-ik dukt] channel that drains lymph from the upper chest and neck

cephalic presentation [seh-FAL-ik pree-zen-TAY-shun] appearance of any part of the fetal head during vaginal delivery

cephalic vein [seh-FAL-ik vayn] a superficial blood vessel that returns blood from the dorsal and palmar surfaces of the forearm to the subclavian vein

-cephalus [sef-uh-lus] *suffix*; head

-ceps [seps] *suffix*; head

cerebellar gait [sair-eh-BEL-ar gayt] a walking stance where the legs are spread widely to compensate for disruption of balance and the tendency to fall

cerebellitis [sair-eh-bel-EYE-tis] inflammation of the cerebellum

cerebellum [sair-eh-BEL-um] a large brain structure located dorsal to the pons and medulla that functions to maintain balance, ocular movement, and posture

cerebral angiography [SER-ee-bral an-jee-OG-ruh-fee] mapping of the cerebral blood vessels using dye and x-rays

cerebral aqueduct [SER-ee-bral AK-weh-dukt] a canal in the midbrain that contains cerebrospinal fluid and connects the third and fourth ventricles

cerebral cortex [SER-ee-bral KOR-teks] outer layer of the cerebrum

cerebral dominance [SER-ee-bral DOM-ih-nants] concept that one hemisphere of the brain exercises greater control or influence for functions such as speech, analytical thinking, mathematics, spatial perception, and motor control

cerebral edema [SER-ee-bral eh-DEE-mah] presence of increased intracranial and extracellular fluid in the white matter of the brain

cerebral palsy [SER-ee-bral PAWL-zee] a group of motor disorders caused by damage to motor centers of the cerebral cortex, cerebellum, or basal ganglia during fetal development, childbirth, or early infancy

cerebral perfusion pressure [SER-ee-bral per-FYOO-zhun PRESH-ur] force needed to ensure that adequate oxygen and nutrients are delivered to tissues

cerebral ventricles [SER-ee-bral VEN-trik-ulz] the four cavities within the cerebrum containing cerebrospinal fluid

cerebrospinal fluid [SER-eh-broh-SPY-nul FLU-id] a fluid secreted by the choroid plexuses of the ventricles of the brain, filling ventricles, subarachnoid spaces, and the spinal cord

cerebrovascular accident [SER-eh-broh-VAS-kyoo-lar AK-si-dent] generalized term pertaining to all strokes without regard to the underlying pathology or mechanism

cerebrum [SER-eh-brum] largest portion of the brain; has left and right hemispheres

cerumen [seh-ROO-men] waxy substance produced by glands in the external auditory meatus which functions to protect the external auditory meatus from infection by trapping microorganisms

ceruminous glands [se-ROO-mih-nus glanz] glands that secrete cerumen or earwax

cervical intraepithelial neoplasia [SER-vi-kal in-trah-ep-ih-THEE-lee-al nee-oh-PLAY-zee-ah] dysplasia of the squamous epithelium of the uterine cervix that may extend into deeper layers

cervical nodes [SER-vih-kal nohdz] lymph nodes located in the neck

cervical plexus [SER-vih-kal PLEKS-us] network of nerves in the cervical region

cervical polyp [SER-vih-kal POL-up] abnormal growth extending from membrane of the cervix uteri

cervical spine [SER-vih-kal spyn] the upper region of the neck consisting of the seven vertebrae

cervical vertebrae [SER-vih-kal VER-te-bray] the seven vertebral segments forming the cervical column in the region of the neck

cervicitis [ser-vik-SIGH-tis] inflammation of the cervix

cervix [SER-viks] the portion of an organ resembling a neck

cervix uteri [SER-viks YOO-ter-eye] the neck of the uterus through which menstrual flow and the fetus pass; structure subject to tears during delivery of a fetus

chalazion [kah-LAY-zee-on] a small, firm, painless lump near the edge of the eyelid, sometimes related to blockage of a meibomian gland

chancre [SHANG-ker] a skin ulcer associated with infection with syphilis

chancroid [SHANG-kroyd] a sexually transmitted infection with *Haemophilus ducreyi* that causes open, painful genital sores

cheilectomy [kye-LEK-toh-mee] surgical removal of osteophytes; the scraping away of bony irregularities

cheilitis [ky-LY-tis] inflammation and cracking of the lips and corners of the mouth due to nutritional deficiency, infection, or allergies

cheiloplasty [KYE-loh-PLAS-tee] surgical repair of the lip, usually because of a laceration

cheilosis [ky-LOH-sis] abnormal condition of the lips characterized by fissures and sores; frequently associated with vitamin B-complex deficiency

chemosis [kee-MO-sis] swelling of the bulbar conjunctiva of the eye that produces swelling around the cornea

chemotaxis [kee-mo-TAK-sis] migration of cells in response to a chemical stimulus

chemotherapy [kee-mo-THER-ah-pee] use of chemical agents to treat disease, especially to treat cancer

cherry hemangioma [CHER-ee he-man-jee-OH-mah] type of birthmark with raised, round tissue comprised of a network of blood vessels

chest physiotherapy [chest fiz-ee-oh-THER-ah-pee] technique of percussing or vibrating the chest wall in an effort to mobilize pulmonary secretions; usually accompanies postural drainage

Cheyne-Stokes respirations [CHAIN-stohks res-pi-RAY-shunz] gradual, transitory respiratory pattern characterized by rapid breathing alternating with periods of apnea, often associated with coma or impending death

chlamydia trachomatis [klah-MID-ee-ah trak-OH-mat-is] the causative organism responsible for sexually acquired disease in the United States

chloasma [kloh-AZ-mah] skin condition associated with pregnancy due to melanocyte-stimulating hormone, characterized by dark hyperpigmentation of the face and a line on the abdomen from pubis to umbilicus called linea nigra

cholangiography [koh-LAN-jee-AWG-rah-fee] process of recording biliary duct function with x-rays

cholecystectomy [koh-lee-sis-TECK-toh-mee] surgical removal of the gallbladder

cholecystic [KOH-lee-SIS-tik] adjective form for gallbladder, pertaining to bile

cholecystitis [koh-lee-sis-TIGH-tis] inflammation of the gallbladder

cholecystogram [koh-ee-SIS-toh-gram] radiological study of the gallbladder and bile ducts

cholecystokinin [KOH-lee-sis-toh-KIN-in] a hormone secreted by the jejunum, duodenum, and hypothalamus that stimulates the release of pancreatic juices and contraction of the gallbadder

cholecystolithiasis [koh-lee-SIS-toh-lih-THIGH-ah-sis] presence of gallstones in the gallbladder

choledochectomy [koh-led-oh-KEK-toh-mee] surgical incision and removal of a portion of the common bile duct

cholelithiasis [koh-lee-lith-AY-uh-sis] gallstones in the gallbladder or bile ducts; attack of abdominal pain caused by colonic spasms

cholestasis [koh-les-TAY-sis] stoppage of the flow of bile, most often due to an obstructive process

cholesteatoma [koh-LES-tee-ah-TOH-mah] a benign, slow-growing mass in the middle ear composed of squamous epithelium and cholesterol deposits that eventually destroys the bones of the middle ear as it invades the mastoid air cells; caused by otitis media

cholesterol [koh-LES-ter-ol] a component of the plasma membrane used to produce bile and steroid hormones (estrogen, progesterone, and testosterone) that can accumulate and deposit abnormally, as in atherosclerosis or gallstones

cholinergics [koh-lin-UR-jiks] drugs that mimic acetylcholine activity to strengthen the esophageal sphincter

cholinesterase inhibitors [koh-lin-ES-ter-ays in-HIB-ih-torz] pharmacological agents that prevent the breakdown of choline at the synapse; used to treat dementia

chondrectomy [kon-DREK-toh-mee] surgical excision of cartilage

chondroblast [KON-droh-blast] immature cartilage cells

chondrodysplasia [kon-droh-dis-PLAY-zee-uh] an inherited growth disorder of bone and cartilage that leads to skeletal malformation and dwarfism

chondroma [kon-DROH-mah] a benign, slow-growing tumor of cartilage

chondromalacia [KON-droh-mah-LAY-shee-ah] softening of the cartilage of a joint

chondrosarcoma [kon-dro-sar-KOH-ma] malignant tumor of cartilage

chordae tendinae [KOR-dee TEN-di-nay] tendinous cords in the heart that look like strings attaching the papillary muscles to the cusps of the mitral and tricuspid valves

chorion [KOH-ree-on] embryonic membrane that makes up part of the placenta

chorionic cavity [koh-ree-ON-ik KAV-ih-tee] space in the extra-embryonic membrane

chorionic villi [koh-ree-ON-ik VIL-eye] vascular projections in the fetal membrane that become the fetal portion of the placenta

chorioretinitis [koh-ree-oh-ret-in-EYE-tis] inflammation of the choroid and retina of the eye

choroid plexus [KO-royd PLEKS-us] structures in the ventricles that secrete cerebral spinal fluid and play a role in intraventricular pressure of the brain

Chron's disease [KRONZ dis-EEZ] an inflammatory bowel disease involving intermittent segments of full thickness of the gastrointestinal tract, occurring most often in the terminal ileum of the small intestine or proximal large intestine; symptoms include abdominal pain, bloody diarrhea, and fistulas

chronic [KRAW-nik] an illness or condition with slow development and long duration, and that persists over a long period of time

chronic obstructive pulmonary disease (COPD) [KRAW-nik ob-STRUK-tive PUL-moe-nar-ee dis-EEZ] lung disorder caused by chronic exposure to irritants such as cigarette smoke and pollution; alveoli rupture creating large spaces and obstruction, characterized by dyspnea, severe productive cough, fatigue, and cyanosis

chronological age [kron-oh-LOJ-ik-al ayj] exact age of a person from birth

chylomicrons [ki-loh-MY-krohz] lipoproteins synthesized in the intestines that transport triglycerides to the liver

chyme [KIME] the semisolid mixture of digestive juices, saliva, and chewed food

chymotrypsin [ky-mo-TRIP-sin] an enzyme secreted by the pancreas that aids in the digestion of protein

cicatrix [SIK-ah-triks] scar tissue that is less elastic, often appears contracted, and lacks normal skin pigmentation

-cidal [sy-dal] *suffix*; to kill

cilia [SIL-ee-ah] small, hairlike projections on the surface of the mucosa that move in waves; singular is cilium

ciliary body [SIL-ee-ar-ee BOD-ee] thickened portion of the vascular tunic of the eye between the choroid and the iris

cingulate gyrus [SIN-gyoo-layt JY-rus] a brain structure with a long, curved convolution on the medial surface of the cortical hemisphere, continuing over the corpus callosum

circa- [sir ka] *prefix*; about

circadian rhythm [sir KAY-dee-ahn RITH-um] physical biorhythms affecting events including body temperature, endocrine function, and sleep cycle

circulatory assist devices [SUR-kyoo-lah-tor-ee ah-SIST dee-VY-sez] instruments that decrease cardiac workload and improve organ perfusion in patients with severe heart failure

circum- [sir-kum] *prefix*; around

circumcision [ser-kum-SIH-zhun] surgical removal of the foreskin or prepuce

circumduction [ser-kum-DUK-shun] movement in which the proximal end is fixed while the distal end moves in a circle

circumflex artery [SER-kum-fleks AR-tur-ee] left vessel that supplies blood to the left atrium and left ventricle

circumoral cyanosis [SER-kum-OR-al SY-ah-NOH-sis] bluish-gray discoloration around the mouth from abnormally low levels of oxygen and abnormally high levels of carbon dioxide in the tissues

circumstantiality [SER-kum-stan-she-AL-ih-tee] a disturbance in thought process evidenced by inclusion of excessive, tangential, and irrelevant information when asked a question; associated with schizophrenia and obsessive disorders

circumvallate papillae [ser-kum-VAL-ayt pa-PIL-aye] circular projections at the back of the tongue containing taste buds

cirrhosis [sir-ROH-sis] inflammation of the liver characterized by nodules and scarring; can be caused by alcoholism, viral hepatitis, or chronic obstruction of the bile ducts

clast- [klast] *prefix*; cell that breaks down substances

claudication [klaw-dih-KAY-shun] modified gait; limping

claustrophobia [KLAW-stroh-FOH-bee-ah] fear of enclosed or small spaces

clavicle [KLAV-ih-kul] a thin, rodlike bone on each side of the anterior neck; commonly referred to as the collarbone

clavus [KLAY-vus] thick, dry callus of skin often occurring on plantar surfaces; also known as a corn

clavus callus [KLAY-vus KAL-us] thickened layer of skin

-cle [kil] *suffix*; small

cleft palate [kleft PAL-at] unilateral or bilateral congenital deformity where the maxilla fails to completely close, resulting in an opening in the bone and skin

clitoris [KLIH-toh-ris] female external genitalia; analogous to the penis

clitoritis [klih-toh-RY-tis] inflammation of the external female genitalia

CLO test (*Campylobacter*-like organism test) [kloh test] a rapid screening test used to detect *Helicobacter pylori* by placing a biopsy of the gastric mucosa on a test pad containing urea; if present, the bacterium changes the urea to ammonia

clonic [KLON-ic] alternating muscular contraction and relaxation; often used to describe seizure activity

-clonus [klon-us] *suffix*; rapid contraction and relaxation

closed fracture [klosd FRAK-shur] a break in which the bone does not penetrate the overlying skin

closed reduction [klosd ree-DUK-shun] medical procedure in which manual manipulation of a displaced fracture is performed so that the bone ends meet to re-establish alignment

clubbing of fingers [KLUB-ing] increased curvature of fingertips due to long-term oxygen supply to the extremities

coarctation of the aorta [koh-ark-TAY-shun uv the ay-OR-tah] congenital narrowing of the aorta, often in the descending aorta near the ductus arteriosus

-coccus [kaw-kus] *suffix*; spherical bacterium

coccygeal [kok-SIJ-ee-al] pertaining to the tailbone or coccyx

coccygeal plexus [kok-SIJ-ee-al PLEK-sus] spinal nerve network in the coccyx region

coccyx [KAWK-siks] tailbone; a group of several small, fused vertebrae that are not individually numbered

cochlea [KOK-lee-ah] a coiled structure located in the inner ear that is shaped like a snail shell and contains the organ of corti

cochlear duct [KOK-lee-ar DUKT] a membranous space inside the cochlea that surrounds the organ of corti

cochlear implant [KOK-lee-ar IM-plant] an amplification device that is surgically inserted into the cochlea in which wires are placed through the round window and into the cochlea

cochleopalpebral reflex [KOK-lee-oh-PAL-peh-bral REE-fleks] contraction of the obicularis palpebrarum muscle in response to sudden loud noise

cognition [kog-NIH-shun] intellectual ability to think including language, calculation, memory, reasoning, and social skill; tested by various neurocognitive screening tools for dementia, depression, and other brain disorders

cognitive-behavioral therapy [KOG-nih-tiv-bee-HAY-vyer-al THAIR-ah-pee] a form of psychotherapy based on the premise that beliefs, attitudes, and thought patterns are learned and can be modified, using various techniques such as guided imagery and self-talk to produce desirable emotions

cogwheel rigidity [KOG-weel ri-JID-ih-tee] stiff, jerky movements of the muscles as if clicking in a gear; associated with Parkinson's disease and side effects of neuroleptic medications

coitus [KO-ih-tus] sexual intercourse

colitis [ko-LYE-tis] an inflammatory condition of the large intestine

collagen [KOL-uh-jen] fibrous protein

collateral ligaments [koh-LAT-er-al LIG-ah-ments] tough, fibrous tissues that provide lateral and medial stability to the knee, ankle, and elbow joints

Colles fracture [KOL-eez FRAK-shur] displacement of the distal end of the radius and ulna

-collis [kol-is] *suffix*; condition of the neck

colloid bath [KOL-oyd bath] immersion in water with dissolved soothing agents to treat skin disorders such as puritis

collum [KOL-um] necklike structure between the head and shoulder

colocolostomy [koh-low-koh-LOS-toe-mee] surgical creation of a new opening between two segments of the colon

colon [KOH-lon] section of the large intestine comprised of the ascending colon, transverse colon, descending colon, and sigmoid colon

colonic [koh-LON-ik] pertaining to the colon

colonic polyposis [ko-LON-ik pol-ee-POE-sis] an inherited condition where large numbers of pendulous growths develop in the mucosa of the colon, with near-certain development of colon cancer; treatment is prophylactic colectomy

colorectal adenocarcinoma [KOH-loh-REK-tal AD-eh-no-KAR-sih-NO-mah] cancerous tumor of the colon caused by colonic polyps or ulcerative colitis that becomes cancerous

colostomy [koh-LOS-toh-mee] surgical creation of an artificial anus on the abdominal wall

colostrum [koh-LOS-trum] liquid that contains protective antibodies secreted by the mammary glands for the few days immediately following childbirth

colpoperineoplasty [KOL-poh-per-ih-NEE-oh-plas-tee] surgical reconstruction of the vagina and perineum

colposcopy [kol-POS-koh-pee] visual examination of the vagina and cervix using an optical magnifying instrument called a colposcope

coma [KO-mah] state of unconsciousness in which the patient cannot be aroused, even with powerful stimuli; may result from trauma, disease, or toxicity

comedo [KOM-ee-doh] accumulation of sebum and keratin in the opening of a hair follicle

comminuted fracture [COM-mih-nyoo-ted FRAK-shur] disruption of the integrity of bone by the bone being crushed into several pieces

commissurotomy [KOM-ih-shur-OT-oh-mee] surgical division of a heart valve due to ventricular hypertrophy

common bile duct [KOM-mon BIHL dukt] the duct formed by the juncture of the cystic and hepatic ducts

communicable [koh-MYOON-ih-kah-bul] capable of being transferred or transmitted to another individual

compound fracture [KOM-pownd FRAK-shur] disruption of the integrity of bone in which the bone breaks through the overlying tissue

compression fracture [com-PRESH-un FRAK-shur] a bone break, especially in a short bone, that disrupts osseous tissue and collapses the affected bone

computerized axial tomography (CAT, CT scan) [kom-PYOO-ter-ized AK-see-al toh-MOG-rah-fee] a radiological procedure that uses x-rays to create images of successive slices of the body and its organs

con- [kon] *prefix*; together or with

conchae [CONG-kay] the three elongated, bony projections known as the superior, middle, and inferior turbinates or nasal conchae; singular is concha

concussion [kon-KUSH-un] brain trauma resulting in transient and/or immediate loss of consciousness due to injury to the soft structure of the brain

condom catheter [CON-dom KATH-eh-ter] an externally applied urinary collection device applied directly to the penis for the management of urinary incontinence

conduction system [kon-DUK-shun SYS-tem] the electrical system of the heart consisting of specialized muscle cells in the right atrium that initiate electrical impulses that spread throughout the heart, causing it to contract

conductive hearing loss [kon-DUK-tiv HEER-ing loss] decreased auditory function caused by a lesion or obstruction of the outer ear

conductive keratoplasty (CK) [kon-DUK-tiv KER-ah-toh-PLAS-tee] surgical procedure to correct farsightedness using heat to shrink tissues around the edge of the cornea to resolve the refractive error

condyle [KON-dyle] articular surface with rounded shape at the end of a bone

condyloid joints [KON-di-loid JOYNTS] articular surfaces in which the oval surface of one bone fits into the elliptical surface of another

condyloma acuminatum [kon-dih-LOH-ma ah-ku-mih-NAH-tum] genital wart due to sexually transmitted disease; plural is condyloma acuminata

cone cells [KOHN sells] cells in the retina of the eye that are sensitive only to color; there are three types of cones: those that respond to red light, those that respond to green light, and those that respond to blue light

congenital [con-JEN-ih-tal] present at birth

congenital dislocation of the hip [con-JEN-ih-tal dis-loh-KAY-shun uv thuh HIP] poor or incomplete formation of the ligaments or acetabulum causing the hip to be loose and not properly functioning

congestive heart failure [kon-JES-tiv hart FAYL-yer] disease in which the heart muscle cannot keep pace to provide the body with oxygenated blood

conjugate gaze [CON-joo-gayt GAYZ] both eyes move together as a unit

conjunctiva [kon-junk-TY-vah] mucous membrane surrounding the eyeball and posterior surfaces of the eyelids; plural is conjunctivae

conjunctivitis [kon-JUNK-tih-VY-tis] inflamed, reddened, and swollen conjunctivae with dilated blood vessels; it has a variety of causes, including foreign substance in the eye, mechanical irritation, or dryness

conjunctivitis, bacterial [kon-JUNK-tih-VY-tis, bak-TEER-ee-al] inflammation and redness of the mucous membrane of the anterior eyeball from bacterial infection; commonly referred to as "pinkeye"

conscious sedation [KON-shus see-DAY-shun] a medically controlled state of depressed consciousness during which the client retains the ability to maintain a continuously patent airway and to respond appropriately to physical stimulation or verbal commands

constipation [CON-stih-PAY-shun] failure to have regular, soft bowel movements

contact dermatitis [KON-takt dur-mah-TYE-tis] skin inflammation caused by an irritant coming in contact with the skin

continuous passive motion machine (CPM) [kon-TIN-yoo-uhs PAS-iv MOH-shun ma-SHEEN] device that increases range of motion and stimulates healing of the articular cartilage by decreasing swelling and the formation of adhesions

continuous positive airway pressure (CPAP) [kon-TIN-yoo-uhs POZ-ih-tiv AIR-way PRESH-ur] a method of keeping the airway open using increased air pressure delivered by a nasal or face mask to treat obstructive sleep apnea, acute pulmonary edema, and congestive heart failure

contra- [kon-tra] *prefix*; opposing or against

contracture [kon-TRAK-chur] condition of fixed resistance to the passive stretch of a muscle; associated with paralysis or lack of use of a muscle group

contraindication [KON-trah-in-dih-KAY-shun] term used in pharmacology to refer a disease or condition that makes the use of certain drugs harmful to the patient

contralateral [kon-trah-LAT-er-al] directional term, pertaining to the opposite side of the body

controlled mandatory ventilation [kon-TROLD MAN-dih-tor-ee ven-tih-LAY-shun] use of a machine to replace and override any impulse to breathe in an intubated patient

contusion [con-TEW-zhun] bruise, bleeding into tissue

convergence [con-VER-jens] medical procedure testing the ability of both eyes to turn medially by holding up an index finger and moving it progressively closer to the patient's nose to test the function of the medial rectus muscles; maximum convergence is called the near point

conversion [con-VER-shun] neurological, sensory, or motor deficits that occur without physical basis; there may be sudden blindness, deafness, paralysis, or inability to speak

convoluted tubule [CON-voh-LEW-ted TOOB-yool] small, twisting tubule in glomerulus in the kidney that connects Bowman's capsule and the loop of Henle

convolutions [kon-voh-LEW-shunz] folds separated by depressions

convulsion [kon-VUL-shun] seizure with a series of sudden, involuntary contractions of muscles of the face, trunk, and extremities

coprolalia [kop-roh-LAY-lee-ah] involuntary verbalizations or gestures that are socially inappropriate, vulgar, obscene, or racist due to Tourette's syndrome

cor pulmonale [KOR pul-mo-NAL-ee] heart disease characterized by right ventricular hypertrophy due to lung disease

coracoid process [KOR-ah-koyd PROS-ess] a small projection that resembles a bent finger; is a point of attachment for several muscles of the arm and chest

cordate [KOR-dayt] having the shape of a heart; can be used to describe heart-shaped tumors

corium [KOH-ree-um] area of skin immediately below the epidermis; also known as dermis

cornea [KOR-nee-ah] the transparent anterior portion of the sclera of the eye

corneal abrasion [KOR-nee-ahl ah-BRAY-shun] loss of or damage to superficial layers of the cornea due to trauma or repetitive irritation, such as a foreign particle under a contact lens

corneal reflex [KOR-nee-al REE-fleks] closing of the eyelid in response to stimulation of the cornea of the eye

corneal transplant [KOR-nee-al TRANZ-plant] grafting a donated cornea to restore function of the eye

corneal ulcer [KOR-nee-al UL-ser] chronic arterial infection and sloughing off of necrotic tissue

coronal plane [kor-OH-nal PLAYN] pertaining to the vertical division of the body into front and back sections

coronary artery disease [KOR-oh-nar-ee AR-ter-ee dis-EEZ] condition in which the myocardium receives inadequate blood supply, pertaining to the heart

coronary bypass [KOR-oh-nar-ee BYE-pass] surgical shunting of heart blood vessels around areas of blockage to restore supply to the heart muscle

coronary circulation [KOR-oh-nar-ee sir-ku-LAY-shun] blood supply to the heart tissue

coronary sinus [KOR-oh-nar-ee SYE-nus] vascular channel draining the coronary veins into the right atrium

corpora cavernosa [COR-por-ah kav-er-NOH-sah] spongy erectile tissues within the penis or clitoris that become engorged during sexual excitation; singular is corpora cavernosum

corpus callosum [KOR-pus kuh-LOH-sum] a broad band of white matter connecting the cerebral hemispheres

corpus spongiosum [KOR-pus spun-jee-OH-sum] erectile tissue that becomes engorged with blood during sexual arousal, causing the penis to become firm and erect; this tissue is located along the underside of the penis

corrugator muscle [KOR-yoo-gay-tor MUS-sel] a facial muscle that draws the eyebrows together to frown

cortex [KOR-teks] the outermost layer of any organ such as a lymph node, kidney, ovary, thymus, or cerebrum

cortical bone [KOR-tih-kal bohn] a superficial, thin layer of compact bone; also called substantia corticalis

cortisol [KOR-ti-sol] hydrocortisone secreted by the adrenal cortex

coryza [ko-RI-za] inflammation of nasal passages associated with profuse nasal discharge, as seen with the common cold

costochondral joint [KOS-toh-KON-dral JOYNT] the area where the costal cartilage meets the bone of the rib

cough [KAWF] forceful exhalation with the intent of clearing the airway of food, fluids, or mucus

counterirritant [kown-ter-IR-ih-tant] a topically applied agent that produces an inflammatory reaction for the purpose of distraction from a primary sensation, usually pain in deeper tissues

coup-contre coup [koo-kon-trah KOO] brain injury with damage occurring on side of impact and on the opposite side of impact due to the forward and backward motion of the brain within the skull

coxa magna [KOK-sah MAG-nah] enlargement of the femoral head causing osteoarthritis of the joint

coxa valga [KOK-sah VAL-gah] deformity of the angle of the femoral neck resulting in outward displacement

coxalgia [kok-SAL-jee-ah] pain in the hip joint

coxarthrosis [koks-ar-THRHO-sis] pain and inflammation of the hip joint due to arthritis

cradle cap [KRAY-del kap] seborrheic dermatitis in infants

cranial [KRAY-nee-al] pertaining to the skull or head

cranial bones [KRAY-nee-al bohnz] osseous structure of the head including the frontal, parietal, temporal, occipital, sphenoid, ethmoid, nasal, vomer, and lacrimal bones, and the inferior nasal concha

cranial nerves [KRAY-nee-al nervs] the twelve paired nerves that emerge from or enter the brain; I: olfactory, II: optic, III: oculomotor, IV: trochlear, V: trigeminal, VI: abducens, VII: facial, VIII: vestibulocochlear, IX: glossopharyngeal, X: vagus, XI: accessory, and XII: hypoglossal

craniectomy [kray-nee-ECK-toh-mee] surgical procedure of opening the skull and removing a portion of the bone

craniosynostosis [KRAY-nee-oh-sin-os-TOH-sis] premature closing of the cranial sutures during the first 18 months of life

cranium [KRAY-nee-um] bony structure that contains the brain

creatinine [kree-AT-in-in] a substance in urine that is found in elevated quantities in patients with muscular dystrophy and other pathologies

Credé method [kre-DAY METH-od] use of external pressure to compress the bladder and express urine when nervous impulses are interrupted

crepitus [KREP-ih-tus] crunching or grinding sounds produced in certain pathological states such as severe arthritis or pneumonia

cretinism [KREE-tin-izm] congenital hypothyroidism that can cause mental retardation if left untreated

Creutzfeldt-Jakob disease [KROITZ-felt-YAH-kop dis-EEZ] progressive fatal neurological disorder caused by an infectious protein particle contracted from cows infected with bovine spongiform encephalopathy

-crine [kreen] *suffix*; secretion of a substance

Crohn's disease (CD) [KROHNZ dis-EEZ] inflammatory bowel disease that can involve any part of the digestive tract; most often found in the ileum, resulting in obstruction of the intestine

cross-section [KROSS-sek-shun] to cut across a plane to study tissue or cells

croup [KROOP] laryngotracheobronchitis in infants and young children caused by bacterial or viral infection of the pharynx in children, characterized by difficult and noisy respiration and a hoarse cough

crusts [KRUSTZ] hard coverings that result when exudate on the skin dries

cry- [kry] *prefix*; cold

cryosurgery [krye-oh-SIR-jir-ee] localized freezing of diseased tissues for surgical removal

cryotherapy [kry-oh-THAIR-ah-pee] use of cold in the treatment of a disease or injury

cryptorchidism [krip-TOR-kih-dizm] failure of one or both testicles to descend

cryptosporidiosis [KRIP-toh-spoh-rid-ee-OH-sis] infection with the protozoa from the genus *Cryptosporidium* that is transmitted through exposure to contaminated food or may be sexually transmitted; typical symptoms are severe diarrhea and abdominal cramps

cuboid [KYOO-boyd] one of the seven bones of the ankle

culdocentesis [kul-doh-sen-TEE-sis] surgical puncture to remove fluid from the cul-de-sac of Douglas

-cule [kule] *suffix*; pertaining to small size

Cullen's sign [KU-lens sine] bluish discoloration around the umbilicus in postoperative clients; can indicate intro-abdominal or perineal bleeding

culture and sensitivity [KUL-chur and SEN-sih-HIV-ih-tee] a laboratory test that utilizes a swab of material from a body part or wound to grow bacteria in culture medium in a Petri dish to identify the infectious agent, then determine which antibiotics are capable of impeding their growth

cuneiform [kyoo-NEE-ih-form] wedge-shaped bones of the hand

curettage [kuu-reh-TAHZH] surgical procedure in which tissue is scraped away using a curette

Cushing's syndrome [KOOSH-ings SIN-drom] a metabolic disorder resulting from the chronic and excessive production of cortisol by the adrenal cortex

Cushing's triad [KOOSH-ings TRY-ad] response associated with increased intracranial pressure or compromised circulation in the brain stem; characterized by hypertension, increased systolic pressure with widened pulse pressure, bradycardia, and irregular respirations

-cusis [kyoo-sis] *suffix*; hearing

-cuspid [kus-pid] *suffix*; points or projections

cutaneous [kyoo-TAY-nee-us] pertaining to or involving the skin

cutaneous papillomas [kyoo-TAY-nee-us pah-pil-OH-mahz] skin tags

cuticle [KEW-ti-kul] fold of skin at the nail root; eponychium

cyan- [sigh-an] *prefix*; blue in color; lacking oxygen

cyanosis [sigh-ah-NOH-sis] bluish skin and mucous membranes resulting from a lack of oxygen in the blood

cycl- [sy-kl] *prefix*; circular; cycle

cycloplegia [sigh-kloh-PLEE-jee-ah] loss of functionality of the ciliary muscle of the eye due to denervation or medication

cycloplegic [sy-klo-PLEE-jik] a pharmacologic agent used to paralyze the ciliary muscle for examination or treatment.

cyclothymia [sigh-kloh-THY-mee-ah] chronic, mild bipolar disorder in which the patient demonstrates mild mood swings with periods of symptom-free intervals for several months

cyst- [syst] *prefix*; pertaining to the urinary bladder or sac

cystic duct [SIS-tik dukt] the duct through which bile from the gallbladder passes into the common bile duct

cystic fibrosis [SIS-tik figh-BROH-sis] an inherited disorder characterized by excessive, thick mucus which causes obstructions in the respiratory and gastrointestinal tract

cystitis [sis-TYE-tis] inflammation of the urinary bladder and ureters resulting from bacterial infection, tumor, or calculus

cystocele [SIS-toh-seel] herniation or protrusion of the urinary bladder into the vagina

cystometerogram [sis-toh-ME-roh-gram] a procedure that measures the bladder dysfunction, most commonly urinary incontinence

cystoplasty [SIS-toh-plas-tee] any reconstructive surgical procedure on the urinary bladder

cystoscopy [sis-TOS-koh-pee] process of visual examination of the urinary bladder using a fiberoptic scope

cystostomy [sis-TOS-toh-mee] creation of a new opening into the urinary bladder for drainage

cystotomy [sis-TOT-oh-mee] incision into the urinary bladder

-cyte [syte] *suffix;* pertaining to a cell

cytology [sy-TOL-oh-jee] study of cells

cytolysis [sy-TOL-ih-sis] destruction of living cells

cytomegalovirus [SY-toh-MEG-ah-loh-VY-rus] a beta-group herpes virus that may be transmitted through sexual or intimate contact that may cause permanent disability, including hearing loss and mental retardation for infants and blindness and mental disorders for adults

cytophotocoagulation [SY-toh-foh-toh-koh-AG-yoo-LAY-shun] destruction of a portion of the ciliary body using an intense beam of light from a laser

cytosol [SY-toh-sol] the liquid portion within the cell membrane

cytotoxic [sigh-toh-TAWK-sik] pharmacological agents or other substances known to be detrimental or destructive to cells

cytotoxin [sigh-toh-TOK-sin] an antibody or other substance that attacks the cells, preventing their normal function and/or destroying them

cyturia [sigh-TUR-ee-ah] presence of any type of cells in the urine

D

dacry- [dak-ree] *prefix*; pertaining to tears

dacryocystitis [DAK-ree-oh-sis-TY-tis] infection of the lacrimal sac of the eye

dacryocystorhinostomy [DAK-ree-oh-SIS-toh-ry-NAWS-toh-mee] surgical procedure that creates a new opening between the lacrimal sac and nose

dacryorrhea [dak-ree-oh-REE-ah] excessive flow of tears; possible causes include inflammation or infection of the eye

dacryostenosis [dak-ree-oh-sten-OH-sis] narrowing of the lacrimal duct due to cysts, tumors, or stone formation

dactyl [DAK-til] a single finger or toe

de- [dee] *prefix*; reversal of, absence

de Lange's syndrome [dee-LANJ SIN-drom] congenital disorder characterized by mental retardation, small head, small stature, generalized failure to thrive, and hirsutism

debridement [day-breed-MOWN] removal of necrotic tissue to foster the regeneration of healthy tissue

decerebrate posturing [dee-SER-eh-brayt POS-chur-ing] physical presentation of rigid extension of the trunk, arms, hands, legs, and feet; associated with lesions of the brain stem

decerebrate rigidity [dee-SER-ee-brayt ri-JID-ih-tee] particular body position caused by a lesion of the upper brain stem; characterized by rigid extension of limbs, internal rotation of the arms, and notable plantar flexion of the feet

decibel (dB) [DES-ih-bel] the intensity of a sound or tone; measurement noted on audiograms and other assessments of hearing

decorticate posturing [dee-KOR-tih-kayt POS-chur-ing] physical sign of pathology in the corticospinal tracts characterized by flexion of the arms and legs

decubitus [dee-KEW-bih-tus] bodily position of lying down

decubitus ulcers [dee-KEW-bit-us UL-surz] skin lesions due to prolonged pressure

deep tendon reflex [deep TEN-don REE-fleks] neurological response to percussion of tendons which produces muscular contraction as demonstrated by the patellar and Achilles reflexes

deep vein thrombosis [deep vayn throm-BOH-sis] blood-clot formation in a deep vein, occurring most frequently in the iliac and femoral veins

defecation [DEF-eh-KAY-shun] process of elimination of end products of digestion by bowel movement

defibrillation [dee-fib-ri-LAY-shun] administration of electrical shock to restore cardiac muscle conduction and contractions

defibrillator [dee-FIB-rih-lay-tor] a medical device that delivers an electric shock to the atria or ventricles of the heart to restore normal heart rhythm; may be an internal or external device

degenerative [dee-JEN-er-ah-tiv] progressive destruction of cells due to disease or aging process

degenerative joint disease (DJD) [dee-JEN-er-ah-tiv JOYNT dis-EEZ] loss of articular cartilage due to aging and cumulative injury to a joint

deglutition [DEE-gloo-TISH-un] the process of swallowing and/or passing food, liquid, or air

dehiscence [dee-HIS-enss] bursting open or splitting of tissue along a natural or sutured line

dehydration [dee-hy-DRAY-shun] state of body water deficit

deleterious [del-ee-TER-ee-us] actions causing injury, harm, or destruction to a patient

delirium [deh-LEER-ee-um] acute confusion, disorientation, and agitation due to toxic levels of body chemicals, drugs, or alcohol in the blood that affect the brain

delirium tremens [deh-LEER-ee-um TREM-enz] caused by withdrawal symptoms from alcoholic intoxication; includes restlessness, tremors of the hands, hallucinations, sweating, and increased heart rate and seizures

delta rhythm [DEL-tah RITH-um] wave pattern on an electroencephalogram typical of deep sleep

delta wave [DEL-tah wayv] premature upstroke of the initial polarization of the heart; a complex of an electrocardiogram finding associated with an atrioventricular bypass tract

deltoid muscle [DEL-toyd MUS-sel] muscle that abducts the upper arm

delusion [dee-LOO-zhun] a fixed false belief that is sustained even when provided evidence to the contrary; due to psychosis or delirium

delusional disorder [dee-LOO-zhun-al dis-OR-der] a psychotic state wherein the patient experiences continued false beliefs despite the efforts of others to persuade or the evidence showing otherwise

dementia [dee-MEN-shee-ah] loss of cognitive and intellectual functioning due to a variety of brain disorders

demineralization [dee-MIN-er-al-ih-ZAY-shun] reduction of minerals such as calcium in body tissues, particularly related to bone

dendrites [DEN-rites] branched nerve fibers carrying impulses toward the cell body

-dendron [den-dron] *suffix*; the branched portion of a nerve cell that receives an impulse

dens [DENZ] a toothlike projection from the second cervical vertebra (C2), upon which the head rotates

deontology [dee-ohn-TOL-oh-jee] a system of ethical decision making that considers the intrinsic moral significance of an action as the basis of decisions

deoxygenated [dee-OKS-eh-jen-aye-ted] without sufficient oxygen

deoxyhemoglobin [dee-OKS-ee-HEE-moh-glo-bin] hemoglobin that is lacking oxygen

depersonalization [dee-PER-son-al-ih-ZAY-shun] loss of connection (dissociative process) between personal thoughts and a sense of self and the environment in which the client reports feeling that he/she is in a dream or watching a movie of him/herself, and things feel unreal and strange; viewing or treating an individual as an object rather than as a person

depigmentation [dee-PIG-men-TAY-shun] white patches of skin due to loss of melanocytes

depolarization [dee-POE-lar-ih-ZAY-shun] the reduction of the membrane potential in nerve or muscle cells to a less negative value

depressed fracture [dee-PREST FRAK-shur] disruption of the cranium where bone is pushed inward toward the brain

depression [dee-PRESH-un] pervasive alteration in mood characterized by low mood, feelings of sadness, social withdrawal, psychomotor retardation, sleep disorder, despair, hopelessness, helplessness, and suicidal thoughts

-derma [derm-uh] *suffix*; skin

dermabrasion [DERM-ah-bray-zhun] dermatological procedure that mechanically scrapes away skin layers

dermagraphism [der-mah-GRAF-izm] condition where hives are produced by scratches or touching the skin

dermatitis [DER-mah-TYE-tis] skin inflammation from any source

dermatoautoplasty [der-mah-toh-AW-toh-plas-tee] skin graft of tissue taken from another area of the patient's body

dermatology [der-mah-TOL-oh-jee] study or treatment of the skin

dermatome [DER-mah-tome] area of skin supplied by a sensory nerve

dermatomyositis [DER-mah-toh-migh-oh-SIGH-tis] inflammation of skin and muscles

dermatophyte [der-MAH-toh-fite] fungal agent that infects the skin, hair, and nails

dermatophytoses [DER-mah-toh-figh-TOH-seez] skin infections caused by fungi

dermis [DER-mis] layer of skin below the epidermis

descending colon [dee-SEN-ding KOH-lon] segment of the small intestine posterior to the splenic flexure and before the sigmoid colon

desensitization [dee-sen-si-ti-ZAY-shun] procedure for making a person insensitive to an antigen; antianaphylaxis

-desis [dee-sis] *suffix*; binding, fuse together

desquamation [des-kwa-MAY-shun] shedding of skin; exfoliation

detrusor muscle [dee-TRU-sor MUS-sel] smooth muscle of the bladder wall

DEXA scan (dual-energy x-ray absorptiometry scan) [DEK-sah scan] a radiological procedure that measures bone mineral density to determine if demineralization from osteoporosis has occurred

dextroscoliosis [DEKS-troh-skoh-lee-OH-sis] an abnormal, excessive, C- or S-shaped lateral curvature of the spine

di- [dye] *prefix*; two

dia- [dy-ah] *prefix*; through, throughout, or completely

diabetes insipidus [dye-ah-BEE-teez in-SIP-ih-dus] chronic pituitary disorder causing antiduretic hormone (ADH) insufficiency

diabetes mellitus [dye-ah-BEE-teez mel-EYE-tus] a metabolic disorder characterized by decreased use of carbohydrates and increased proteins and lipids due to absence of insulin production

diabetes mellitus, type I [dye-ah-BEE-teez mel-EYE-tus] juvenile diabetes characterized by destruction of insulin producing beta cells of the islets of Langerhans in the pancreas; possible etiologies include genetic inheritance and viral infection that triggers an autoimmune response

diabetes mellitus, type II [dye-ah-BEE-teez mel-EYE-tus] condition in which the body produces insufficient insulin, or defective use of insulin produced; treatment includes oral agents, insulin if needed, dietary restriction, and weight loss

diabetic ketoacidosis (DKA) [DYE-ah-BET-ik KEE-toh-AS-ih-DOH-sis] in uncontrolled diabetes and starvation, an abnormal utilization of carbohydrates results in excessive production of ketone bodies during oxidation of fatty acids

diabetic neuropathy [DYE-ah-BET-ik nyoo-ROP-ah-thee] damage to peripheral nerves of the lower legs and feet due to poorly controlled blood glucose levels

diabetic retinopathy [DYE-ah-BET-ik ret-ih-NAWP-ah-thee] condition associated with long-standing diabetes; characterized by damage to the retina of the eye by interrupted vascularization from hemorrhages, micro-aneurysms, and waxy deposits

diagnosis [dye-ag-NOE-sis] identification of a pathological state or disorder

dialysis [dye-AL-ih-sis] artificial procedure used to replace normal kidney filtering by using an external filtration system

diaphoresis [dye-uh-foh-REE-sis] profuse sweating

diaphragm [DYE-ah-fram] a curved, muscular membrane that divides the thoracic and abdominal cavities

diaphysis [dy-AF-ih-sis] the midsection or shaft of a long cylindrical bone, such as the femur

diarrhea [DYE-ah-REE-uh] abnormally frequent and loose, watery stools with increased peristalsis caused by an infection (bacteria, viruses), irritable bowel syndrome, ulcerative colitis, lactose intolerance, or a drug side effect

diastole [dye-AS-toh-lee] relaxation of the heart, allowing it to refill with blood for the next contraction

diastolic blood pressure [dye-us-TOL-ik BLUD presh-ur] force exerted by the circulating blood on the arterial walls during ventricular relaxation and filling

diathermy [DYE-ah-therm-ee] therapeutic use of electromagnetic ultrasound waves to heat muscle tissue

diencephalon [dye-en-CEF-uh-lon] brain structure containing the thalamus and hypothalamus

diffusion [di-FYOO-zhun] movement of molecules in a solution or a gas from an area of high concentration to one of low concentration

digital subtraction angiography [DIJ-ih-tahl sub-TRAK-shun an-jee-OGH-rah-fee] computerized imaging of the vasculature with visualization on a monitor screen following the intravenous injection of iodine through a catheter

digitalis [dij-ih-TAL-is] a pharmacological agent that increases the strength of heart muscle contraction

digitalization [dij-ih-tal-ih-ZAY-shun] administration of a larger loading dose of digitalis to speed therapeutic response without producing toxic symptoms

dilated funduscopy [DIH-layt-ed fun-DOS-kohp-ee] procedure to examine the posterior cavity using mydriatic eyedrops to dilate the pupil (a process known as cycloplegia)

dilation and curettage [dye-LAY-shun and kuh-reh-TAJH] dilation of the cervix and scraping of the endometrium

dilation and extraction [dye-LAY-shun and eks-TRAK-shun] dilation of the cervix and removal of the products of conception

diplegia [di-PLEE-jee-ah] paralysis involving both arms or both legs

diplococcus [dip-loh-KOK-us] spherical or oval-shaped bacterium, occurring in pairs; plural is diplococci

diplopia [dih-PLOH-pee-ah] visual disturbance where single objects are perceived as two objects; caused by increased intracranial pressure or by multiple sclerosis that affects nerve conduction

-dipsia [dip-see-uh] *suffix*, thirst

dis- [dys] *prefix*; away from

disc [DISK] small, circular bone with two flat surfaces; acts as a cushion to decrease impact during body movements

discoid lupus erythematosus [DYS-koid LOO-pus er-ih-thee-mah-TOH-sus] autoimmune disease of connective tissue

dislocation [dis-loh-KAY-shun] displacement of the end of a bone from its normal position within a joint; usually caused by injury or trauma

dismember [dis-MEM-ber] to remove an arm or leg by surgical amputation

disorganized schizophrenia [dis-OR-gan-izd skitz-oh-FRE-nee-ah] a severe thought disorder characterized by incoherent thought processes, inappropriate affect, silly and childlike mannerisms, but without delusions

disorientation [DIS-ore-ee-en-TAY-shun] loss of information as to person, date, time, surroundings, and situation; caused by acute illness or dementia

displaced fracture [dis-PLAYSD FRAK-chur] when broken bone ends are pulled out of their normal anatomical alignment

dissecting aneurysm [dys-SEK-ting AN-yoo-riz-um] bulge or tear occurring between the arterial walls due to blood forcing its way through a tear in the intima between the arterial layers

dissection [dih-SEK-shun] surgical removal or extensive incision

disseminated [dih-SEM-ih-nay-ted] condition of wide dispersement throughout an tissue, organ, or body part

disseminated intravascular coagulation [dih-SEM-ih-nay-ted IN-tra-VAS-kyoo-lar koh-ag-yoo-LAY-shun] disruption of clotting due to hyperstimulation of coagulation pathways resulting in unfocused clotting action that exhausts necessary clotting factors such that generalized and severe bleeding occurs

dissociated nystagmus [dih-SOH-see-ayt-ed nis-TAG-mus] rhythmic movements of the eyes where the movements differ in directions, rate, and severity

dissociative fugue [dih-SOH-see-ah-tiv FEWG] impulsive flight from one's life and familiar surroundings following a traumatic event; the patient begins a new life in a new location and functions normally without recall of the past

dissolution [dih-soh-LEW-shun] rate at which a drug becomes a solution

dista equinus [DIS-tah ek-QWEE-nus] limited ability to dorsiflex the foot; associated with clubfoot

distal [DYS-tal] away from the center or point of origin

distal interphalangeal joint (DIP) [DYS-tal in-ter-fah-LAN-jee-ahl joynt] the articular surface between the last two phalanges in a finger or toe

distribution [dis-tri-BYOO-shun] movement of drugs from the blood into various body liquids and tissues

distributive shock [dis-TRIB-yoo-tiv shok] abnormal pooling of blood in the extremities due to anaphylaxis, sepsis, or spinal cord injury

diuresis [dye-yoo-REE-sis] increased urine formation and secretion

diuretics [dye-yoo-RET-iks] pharmacological agents that increase urinary output

diurnal [dy-YUR-nal] pertaining to a daily occurrence of body rhythms, such as circadian rhythm

diverticulitis [DYE-ver-TIK-yoo-LYE-tis] feces become trapped inside a diverticular sac, resulting in inflammation and infection, abdominal pain, and fever

diverticulosis [dy-ver-tik-yoo-LOH-sis] formation of pouches in the wall of the colon, usually without inflammation

diverticulum [DYE-ver-TIK-yoo-lum] area of the intestinal surface where the mucosa has been forced out through small defects in the wall of the colon

divulsor [dih-VUL-sor] a medical tool used to dilate a body part, such as the urethra

dopamine [DOHP-ah-meen] neurotransmitter in the brain

Doppler [DOP-lur] determination of blood flow; velocity, direction, and possible occlusion using a transducer placed over the blood vessel; data obtained is analyzed by computer for pathology

dorsal [DOR-sal] pertaining to back part

dorsal column [DOR-sal KOL-lum] white matter in the posterior region of the spinal cord that contains motor neurons

dorsal horn [DOR-sal horn] horn-shaped projection of gray matter in the posterior region of the spinal cord

dorsal muscles [DOR-sal MUS-selz] skeletal muscles of the back including the trapezius and latissimus dorsi

dorsal ramus [DOR-sal RAY-mus] branch of spinal nerves that passes on the back surface to innervate skin, muscle, and bones of the vertebral column

dorsal recumbent [DOR-sal rih-KUM-bent] position of a patient lying down on the back, with the face up

dorsal reflex [DOR-sal REE-fleks] involuntary contraction of the muscles of the back in response to irritation of the skin over the erector spinae muscles

dorsal root [DOR-sal root] sensory nerve fibers of the spinal cord

dorsal root ganglion [DOR-sal root GANG-lee-on] a mass of nerve tissue containing the cell bodies of sensory neurons that is located on the dorsal surface of the nerve root

dorsalis pedis [dor-SAL-is PEE-dis] pulse found on the top surface of the foot

dorsiflexion [dor-si-FLEK-shun] movement of a body part in toward the center and upward

dorsodynia [dor-soh-DIN-ee-ah] pain in the upper muscles of the back

-dose [dohs] *suffix*; measured quantity or amount

-drome [drohm] *suffix*; running

duct [DUKT] an open channel through which secretions or other substances pass

ductus arteriosus [DUK-tus ar-TEER-ee-OH-sus] an oval opening in the septum between the atria in the heart that exists before birth and closes at birth, when breathing begins

ductus deferens [DUK-tus DEF-er-enz] a long, narrow tube that receives spermatozoa from the epididymis; also known as the vas deferens

dumping syndrome [DUMP-ing SIN-drom] physical effects of rapid gastric motility following gastric surgery; these effects include diaphoresis, tachycardia, the urge to lie down, diarrhea, and dehydration in severe cases; relieved by frequent small meals without liquids

duodenal [DOO-OD-eh-nal] pertaining to the duodenum

duodenocholangitis [dyoo-OD-en-oh-koh-lan-JYE-tis] inflammation of the duodenum and common bile duct

duodenorrhaphy [dyoo-oh-deh-NOR-ah-fee] suturing of the duodenum

duodenum [DOO-oh-den-um] a 10-inch-long section of bowel that immediately follows the stomach and connects with the jejunum

dura mater [DYOO-rah MAH-ter] the tough, fibrous membrane that forms the outermost covering of the central nervous system

dyad [DIE-ad] a pair, or two people in an interaction; often used to describe a mother-and-newborn interaction

-dynia [dye-nee-ah] *suffix*; painful

dys- [dis] *prefix*; faulty, painful, difficult, or abnormal

dysarthria [dis-AR-three-uh] difficulty forming clear speech due to dysfunction of the throat muscles

dysboulia [dis-BYOO-lee-ah] difficulty focusing on a task; poor concentration or thinking ability

dyschromia [dys-KROH-mee-uh] abnormal color of skin due to disease, radiotherapy, or cytotoxic drugs

dysconjugate [dis-CON-joo-gayt] condition in which the eyes do not move in tandem

dyscrasia [dis-KRAY-zee-ah] blood-related diseases affecting blood cells or platelets

dysentery [DIS-en-tair-ee] bacterial infection caused by an unusual strain of *E. coli* bacterium in the large intestine; symptoms include watery diarrhea mixed with blood and mucus

dysesthesia [dys-es-THEE-zee-uh] perception of an irritating sensation in response to normal stimuli due to nerve dysfunction

dyskinesia [dis-ki-NEE-zee-ah] experiencing difficulty in performance of voluntary movements

dyslogia [dis-LOH-jee-ah] impaired speech and reasoning due to a mental disorder

dysmenorrhea [dys-men-oh-REE-ah] painful menstruation

dyspareunia [dis-pah-RYOO-nee-uh] painful sexual intercourse

dyspepsia [dis-PEP-see-ah] indigestion or epigastric pain that may be accompanied by gas or nausea; possibly caused by excess secretion of stomach acid, overeating, spicy foods, or stress

dysphagia [dis-FAY-jee-ah] difficulty swallowing

dysphonia [dis-FOH-nee-ah] difficulty producing speech with regard to sound quality and pronunciation

dysphoria [dis-FOR-ee-ah] generally unhappy mood, depression, and anxiety

dysplasia [dis-PLAY-zee-ah] abnormal growth and development of tissue

dyspnea [disp-NEE-uh] difficulty breathing or shortness of breath

dysrhythmia [dis-RITH-mee-ah] irregular heart rhythm, rate, or sequence of cardiac activation

dysthymia [dis-THY-mee-ah] chronic, mild to moderate depression

dystocia [dis-TOE-see-ah] difficult childbirth due to large fetal size, small pelvic outlet, or malpositioning of the fetus, such as breech presentation

dystonia [dis-TOH-nee-ah] state of hyper- or hypotonicity of tissue; most often used in reference to muscle tone

dysuria [dis-YOO-ree-ah] pain during urination, often caused by infection, irritation, or obstruction of the urinary tract

E

e- [ee] *prefix*; without, absent; away from or outside

-eal [eel] *suffix*; pertaining to

ec- [ek] *prefix*; out or away from

ecchymosis [EK-ih-MOH-sis] large hemorrhages or bruises on the skin

eccrine [EK-rin] denoting the flow of sweat

echocardiogram [ek-oh-KAHR-dee-oh-gram] image of the heart produced by ultrasound

echogenic [ek-oh-JEN-ik] characteristic of body tissues that resonate echoes of sound which are captured under ultrasound examination

echolalia [EK-oh-LAY-lee-ah] disorder of speech associated with schizophrenia where the patient automatically repeats (echoes) what someone else has said

-ectasis [ek-tay-sis] *suffix;* dilation or expansion

ecto- [ek-toh] *prefix;* outside

ectogenous [ek-TOJ-eh-nus] conditions produced from sources outside of the body; disease that is caused by events outside the body such as infections or traumatic injury

-ectomy [ek-toh-mee] *suffix;* to cut, excise, or remove

ectopic [ek-TOP-ik] malplacement of an organ or an object; for example, an ectopic pregnancy, which occurs outside of the uterus—or an event such as a heartbeat

ectropion [ek-TROH-pee-on] weakening of connective tissue in the lower eyelid in older patients causing the eyelid to turn outward, exposing the conjunctiva and causing dryness and chronic conjunctivitis

eczema [EK-ze-mah] genetic inflammatory skin disorder

edema [eh-DEE-mah] swelling of a body part

edentulous [ee-DEN-tyoo-lus] lacking natural teeth

efferent [EF-er-ent] conduction or activity moving outward

efferent lymphatic vessel [EF-er-ent lym-FAT-ik VES-sel] a structure that carries lymph toward the periphery

efferent nerve [EF-er-ent nerv] a peripheral nerve that conveys impulses from the central nervous system to the peripheral nerves; opposite of an afferent nerve

effusion [ee-FYOO-zhun] accumulation of fluid

egesta [ee-JEST-ah] the unabsorbed food fragments that are passed through the digestive tract

ejaculation [ee-JAK-yoo-LAY-shun] series of contractions producing emission of 2–5 mL of semen from the male urethra

ejaculatory [ee-JAK-yoo-lah-tor-ree] pertaining to the emission of semen from the male urethra

ejaculatory duct [ee-JAK-yoo-la-tor-ee dukt] the passage formed by the junction of the duct of the seminal vesicles and ductus deferens through which semen enters the urethra

ejection fraction [ee-JEK-shun FRAK-shun] the percentage of blood emptied from the ventricle during contraction; normal value for healthy hearts is 60–70 percent but may be much lower with valve disorders or myocardial infarction

ejection murmur [ee-JEK-shun MUR-mur] an abnormal cardiac sound produced by pumping of blood into the aorta or pulmonary arteries that stops prior to the closure of the aortic or pulmonic valves

elasticity [ee-las-TIS-ih-tee] demonstrating the ability to stretch

electroanalgesia [ee-lek-troh-an-al-JEE-zee-ah] use of electrical stimulation to compete with pain stimuli for transmission to the spinal cord; may be delivered through the skin or by an implantable device

electrocardiogram [ee-lek-troh-KAHR-dee-oh-gram] record of the electrical forces producing heart contractions

electrocochleography [ee-LEK-troh-kok-lee-OG-rah-fee] process of recording the electrical activities of the cochlea of the inner ear

electroconvulsive therapy (ECT) [ee-LEK-troh-con-VUL-siv THAIR-ah-pee] use of electrical current and electrodes on the head to produce seizures while sedated; alters the brain chemistry to treat severe depression more rapidly than antidepressant drugs

electrodesiccation [ee-LEK-troh-des-ih-kay-shun] use of an electrode to apply high-frequency, short electrical currents to destroy tissue by drying

electroencephalogram [ee-LEK-troh-en-SEF-ah-loh-grahm] graphic recording of the brain's electrical activity

electroencephalograph [ee-LEK-troh-en-SEF-ah-loh-graf] an instrument used to record the electrical activity of the brain

electrolarynx [ee-LEK-troh-LAR-inks] an external device applied to the throat to amplify breath sounds in patients following surgical removal of the larynx

electrolysis [ee-lek-TROL-ih-sis] destruction of tissue by electric current

electrolytes [ee-LEK-troh-lites] soluble, inorganic ions, such as sodium and chloride, found in body fluids

electromyography [ee-LEK-troh-migh-OG-rah-fee] record of muscular activity for diagnostic purposes using electrodes

electron [ee-LEK-tron] a negatively charged subatomic particle

electrophoresis [ee-LEK-troh-for-EE-sis] movement of particles within an electric field toward a cathode or anode

elephantiasis [el-eh-fan-TYE-ah-sis] massive swelling of the lower extremities or genitalia; also called pachydermas

elimination [ee-LIM-ih-nay-shun] process of removal of undigested and residual liquids from the body

elytro- [el-eye-troh] *prefix*; pertaining to the vagina

emaciation [ee-may-see-AY-shun] excessive leanness earned by muscle wasting

embolectomy [em-boh-LEK-toh-mee] removal of a clot from a blood vessel by surgical or enzymatic methods

embolism [EM-boe-lizm] mass of undissolved matter present in a blood or lymphatic vessel brought there by the blood or lymph current

embolization [em-bol-ih-ZAY-shun] formation and release of a substance to occlude blood vessels in the treatment or prevention of hemorrhaging

embolotherapy [em-boh-loh-THAIR-ah-pee] intentional obstruction of the lumen of a blood vessel by injection of a solution or dislodgement of thrombus or plaque

embolus [EM-bow-lus] substance or mass that stops the flow of a vessel

embryology [em-bree-OL-oh-jee] study of the origin and development of a fetus from fertilization up to the time of birth

embryonic stage [em-bree-ON-ik STAJ] developmental stage that occurs during the first 2–8 weeks after fertilization of a human egg

emesis [EM-eh-sis] expelled food or chyme

-emesis [em-ee-sis] *suffix*; vomiting

emetic [ee-MET-ik] an agent that causes vomiting

-emia [ee-muh] *suffix*; blood condition

-emic [ee-mik] *suffix*; pertaining to the blood or substance in blood

emmetropia [em-eh-TRO-pee-ah] normal vision

emphysema [em-fih-SEE-mah] chronic and irreversible damage to alveoli characterized by trapped air in the lung; productive cough, often due to smoking or pollution

empyema [em-pye-EE-mah] presence of pus in a bodily cavity; used most often in reference to pyothorax

emulsification [ee-MUL-si-fi-kay-shun] process of breaking down large globules of fats into smaller particles

en- [en] *prefix*; in

-ence [ens] *suffix*; state of

encephalitis [en-sef-ah-LYE-tis] inflammation of the brain due to bacterial or viral infection

encephalocele [en-SEF-ah-loh-seel] protrusion or herniation of the brain and meninges

encephalomalacia [en-SEF-ah-loh-mah-LAY-sha] softening of the brain due to ischemia or infarction

encephalomyelopathy [en-SEF-ah-loh-mye-LOH-path-ee] disease that affects both the brain and spinal cord

encephalopathy [en-sef-ah-LOP-ah-thee] cerebral dysfunction due to an insult to the brain such as a toxin, injury, inflammation, or anoxic event

encephalosclerosis [en-SEF-ah-loh-skle-ROH-sis] hardening of the brain, especially the cerebrum, due to plaque formation or hypertension

encopresis [en-koh-PREE-sis] repeated passage of stool into the clothing in a child older than age five in the absence of gastrointestinal illness or disability

end- [end] *prefix*; within or inside

endarterectomy [end-art-er-EK-toh-mee] surgical excision of fatty deposits along with diseased endothelium and significant portions of the arterial lining

endo- [en-doh] *prefix*; within or inside

endocardium [en-doh-KAR-dee-um] the lining of the heart chambers

endocrine system [EN-doh-krin SIS-tem] structures within the body that are capable of secreting hormones; includes the hypothalamus, pituitary gland, thyroid gland, pancreas, testis, ovaries, adrenal glands, thymus, parathyroid glands, and pineal gland

endocrinology [EN-doh-krin-OL-oh-jee] the study of the endocrine system

endogenous [en-DOJ-eh-nus] disease that originates from factors inside the body; for example, autoimmune disorders

endolymph [EN-doh-lymf] liquid within the membranous labyrinth of the inner ear

endometriosis [en-doh-mee-tree-OH-sis] presence of endometrial tissue at sites other than the uterus

endometritis [en-doh-mee-TRY-tis] inflammation of the endometrium (lining of the uterus) due to bacterial infection

endometrium [en-doh-MEE-tree-um] the innermost layer of the uterine wall

endomysium [en-doh-MYZ-ee-um] the sheath of connective tissue that surrounds each muscle fiber

endoneurium [en-doh-NOO-ree-um] connective tissue surrounding an individual nerve fiber

endopericarditis [EN-doh-per-ee-kar-DY-tis] inflammation of the endocardium and pericardium of the heart

endoplasm [EN-doh-plazm] the portion of the cell between the cell membrane and nucleus that contains the cellular organelles

endoplasmic reticulum [en-doh-PLAS-mik reh-TIK-yoo-lum] a network of microscopic channels or tubes extending throughout the cytoplasm that serves as a transport system for materials within the cell

endoscope [EN-doh-skope] an instrument used to examine the interior of the body

endoscopic retrograde cholangiopancreatography [en-doh-SKOP-ik RET-roh-grade ko-LAN-jee-oh-pan-KREE-ah-toh-grah-fee] use of a fiberoptic scope to examine the pancreatic, bile, and hepatic ducts followed by injection of a contrast medium for radiography of the biliary and pancreatic ducts

endoscopic sonography [en-doh-SKOP-ic soh-NOG-rah-fee] examination of internal tissues or structures by placing a transducer inside body cavity to produce images by conduction of sound waves

endotoxin [en-doh-TOK-sin] a poisonous substance in the walls of gram-negative bacteria that produces a systemic inflammatory response and sepsis

endotracheal [EN-doh-TRAY-kee-al] pertaining to the innermost aspect of the trachea

endotracheal intubation [en-doe-TRAY-kee-al in-tyoo-BAY-shun] passage of a tube into the trachea through the nose or mouth to open the airway for delivery of air, oxygen, or anesthesia

end-stage renal disease [end-stayj REE-nal dis-EEZ] final phase of kidney disease marked by the inability to filter the body's blood

-ent [ent] *suffix*; person or agent

enteral nutrition [EN-ter-ahl nu-TRI-shun] delivery of nutrients through a gastrointestinal tube or other artificial means

enterobiasis [en-ter-oh-BY-ah-sis] pinworm infestation of the large intestine

enterocolectomy [EN-ter-oh-koh-LEK-toh-mee] surgical excision of the terminal ileum, cecum, and ascending colon

enterocolitis [EN-ter-oh-koh-LY-tis] inflammation of the small bowel due to bacterial or viral infection; possible causative agents include rotaviruses, *Campylobacter*, *Escherichia coli*, and *Salmonella* bacterial species

enterospasm [EN-ter-oh-SPAZM] sudden, involuntary, painful contraction of intestinal muscles

enterotomy [en-ter-OT-oh-mee] surgical incision into the small intestine

-entery [en-ter-ee] *suffix*; condition of the intestine

entodynia [en-toh-DYE-nee-ah] intestinal pain

entropion [en-TROH-pee-on] weakening of the muscle in the lower eyelid, occurring most often in older adults

enucleation [ee-nyoo-klee-AYE-shun] surgical procedure to remove the entire structure of the eye from the orbit due to trauma or a tumor

enuresis [en-yoo-REE-sis] involuntary nighttime bed-wetting, particularly in children

environmental disease [en-VY-rawn-MEN-tal dis-EEZ] illness associated with or due to external substances

enzyme [EN-zime] chemical substance produced by the body's endocrine system or organs to break down large molecules into smaller components for digestion; often ends with the *suffix* -ase

ependymoma [ep-en-dye-MOH-mah] brain neoplasm tumor derived from ependymal cells

epi- [ep-ih] *prefix*; upon, surface, or above

epicardium [ep-ih-KAHR-dee-um] outer heart layer; membranous lining of the inner heart

epicondylitis [EP-ih-kon-dih-LY-tis] inflammation of the elbow joint at the point of the articular surfaces of the humerus

epicranius muscle [ep-ee-KRAY-nee-us MUS-sel] muscle that raises eyebrows, as demonstrated by the expression of surprise

epidemic [ep-ih-DEM-ik] occurrence of a disease in greater-than-expected proportion over a geographic region

epidemiology [EP-ih-dee-mee-OL-oh-jee] study of the distribution and determinants of health-related states or events in populations

epidermis [ep-ih-DER-mis] outermost, superficial skin layer

epidermolysis [ep-ih-DER-moh-LIE-sis] separation of the dermal and epidermal layers of skin

epididymis [ep-ih-DID-ih-mis] a long, coiled duct that carries sperm from the seminiferous tubules of the testes to the vas deferens

epididymitis [EP-ih-did-ih-mye-tis] acute or chronic inflammation of the epididymis resulting from a variety of conditions, including urinary tract infection, venereal disease, prostatitis, or prolonged use of indwelling urinary catheters

epididymoorchitis [ep-ih-di-dye-MOOR-ky-tis] inflammation of the testes and the epididymis

epigastric [EP-ih-GAS-trik] abdominal region between the tip of the sternum and above the umbilicus

epigastric tamponade [EP-ih-GAS-trik tam-pon-AYD] insertion of a tampon or plug in the epigastric region to control bleeding

epiglottic [EP-ih-GLOT-ik] pertaining to the epiglottis

epiglottis [EP-ih-GLOT-is] a valvelike structure in the throat that seals off the larynx or airway, shunting food, saliva, and other liquids into the esophagus

epiglottitis [EP-ih-glot-TYE-tis] severe infection or inflammation of the epiglottis and surrounding tissues which can result in stridor, respiratory distress, and partial to complete airway obstruction; occurs most commonly in children ages 2–12

epihyal [ep-ih-HIE-yal] pertaining to the arch of the hyoid bone at the base of the tongue

epilepsy [EP-ih-lep-see] disorder affecting the central nervous system; characterized by recurrent seizures

epinephrine [ep-ih-NEF-rin] adrenal medulla hormone; adrenaline

epineurium [ep-ih-NEW-ree-um] connective tissue around a nerve trunk

epiphyseal line [ee-PIF-ih-seel lyn] the closed border of the growth plate at the end of a bone when it has stopped growing

epiphyseal plate [eh-PIF-ih-seel playt] a disc of cartilage located between the epiphysis and the metaphysis of long bones during growth

epiphysis [ee-PIF-ih-sis] the bulbous portion of bone located at the proximal and distal ends of long bones; plural is epiphyses

epiphysis cerebri [eh-PIF-ih-sis SER-eh-brye] pineal gland; a cone-shaped organ in the brain that secretes melatonin

episiorrhaphy [eh-piz-ee-OR-ah-fee] suturing of the vulva and perineum

episiotomy [eh-piz-ee-OT-oh-mee] process of cutting the vulva; used to assist delivery of the fetus

epispadias [ep-ih-SPAY-dee-us] congenital defect in which the urethral opening is located on the penis dorsum in males and the clitoris in females

epithelial root [ep-ih-THEE-lee-al root] nail part beneath the cuticle

epithelium [ep-ih-THEE-lee-um] cellular layer that forms the epidermis of the skin and outermost surface of the serous mucous membranes

eponychium [ep-OH-nik-ee-um] fold of skin near the nail root

equi- [ek-wee] *prefix*; equal, as in size or distance

equianalgesic [EK-wah-an-al-JEE-sik] the amount of a drug required, whether administered orally or parenterally, needed to produce the same analgesic effect when changing from one formulation to another

equivocal [ee-QUIV-oh-kul] questionable, doubtful, or vague

Erb palsy [erb PAWL-zee] paralysis of the upper arm and shoulder due to a lesion of the upper trunk of the brachial plexus or the fifth and sixth cervical roots

erector spinae muscles [ee-REK-tor SPY-nee MUS-selz] muscular group of the dorsal spine that originates at the sacrum, ilium, and lumbar vertebrae and attaches at the ribs and upper thoracic vertebra; the function is to maintain upright posture and extend the vertebral column

erotomania [ER-oh-toh-MA-nee-ah] pathological preoccupation with erotic ideas and behavior; delusional belief that the patient is romantically involved with a celebrity or desirable person; associated with acute mania and schizophrenia

erysipelas [er-ih-SIP-ee-las] acute cellulitis of the skin

erythema [er-ih-THEE-ma] redness on the skin

erythroblastosis fetalis [eh-RITH-row-blas-TOW-sis fee-TAL-is] hemolytic disorder of a newborn characterized by jaundice, anemia, generalized edema, and enlargement of the spleen and liver

erythrocytosis [eh-RITH-roh-sye-TOE-sis] abnormally increased amount of red blood cells in circulation; associated with hypoxemia and polycythemia vera

erythropoiesis [eh-RITH-roh-poy-EE-sis] production of red blood cells

erythropoietin [eh-rith-roh-POY-eh-tin] a glycoprotein hormone released into the bloodstream in response to hypoxia which increases the production of red blood cells; also a hormone secreted by the kidney that stimulates the bone marrow to produce red blood cells

eschar [ES-kar] thick scar that forms over a healed burn

Escherich's reflex [ESH-er-iks REE-fleks] involuntary muscular contraction of the mouth when the mucosa of the lips is stimulated; this is noted particularly in newborns

-esis [ee-sis] *suffix;* condition or state of being

esophageal [ee-SOF-ah-JEE-al] pertaining to the esophagus

esophageal sphincter [ee-SOF-ah-JEE-al SFINK-ter] valve at the end of the esophagus as it joins with the stomach that prevents reflux of gastric contents into the esophagus

esophageal varices [ee-SOF-ah-JEE-al VAR-ih-seez] twisted, swollen veins in the esophagus

esophagitis [ee-SOF-ah-JY-tis] chronic inflammation of the esophagus; this inflammation can progress to esophageal ulcers or cancer of the esophagus

esophagospasm [ee-SOF-ah-goh-spazm] sudden, involuntary, often painful contraction of the muscles of the esophagus

esophagus [ee-SOF-ah-gus] a flexible, muscular tube leading from the pharynx to the stomach

esotropia [es-oh-TROH-pee-ah] turning inward of the eyeball

esterase [ES-ter-ace] an enzyme that splits organic compounds such as fats

estra- [es-trah] *prefix*; outside of

estradiol [es-trah-DEE-ohl] a naturally occurring estrogen that is formed by the ovary, placenta, testes, and adrenal cortex

estrogen [ES-troh-jen] hormones secreted by the placenta, and in small amounts by the adrenal cortex; responsible for many female reproductive functions, including secondary female characteristics

ethmoid bone [ETH-moyd bohn] bone forming the anterior base of the cranium, bony nasal septum, and medial walls of the eye sockets

ethmoid sinuses [ETH-moyd SIGH-nus-ez] one of the air chambers within the ethmoid bone

etiology [ee-tee-AWL-oh-jee] underlying cause of a disorder

eu- [yoo] *prefix*; normal or good

eucrasia [yoo-KRA-see-ah] state of normal health with balance in all activities or processes

eupnea [YOOP-nee-ah] breathing with normal depth and rate

eury- [yur-ee] *prefix*; broad or thickened

eustachian tube [yoo-STAY-shun toob] a small canal between the inner ear and throat that allows air pressure in the middle ear to equalize with air pressure in the mouth and outside the body

eustress [YOO-stress] a type of stress that results in positive change or growth

eutocia [yoo-TOE-see-uh] normal labor

eversion [ee-VER-shun] turning a body part outward

evoked potentials [ee-VOKT poh-TEN-shalz] stimulation of the central nervous system by stimulation of a sensory nerve which is recorded in an electroencephalogram

Ewing's sarcoma [YOO-ingz sar-KOH-mah] a malignancy of the bones of the extremities and shoulder girdle, with a typical onset before age 20

ex- [eks] *prefix*; out or away from, external

exacerbation [eks-az-er-BAY-shun] increase in symptoms or severity of disease

excisional biopsy [ek-SIH-zhun-al BY-op-see] removal of an entire suspected lesion for microscopic examination

excoriation [eks-koh-ree-AY-shun] skin abrasion

excrete [eks-KREET] to move substances produced within endogenous tissues and organs out of the body

excretory cystogram [EKS-cree-tor-ee SIS-toh-gram] a radiographic examination of excretory organs

excretory urogram [EKS-cree-tor-ee YOO-roh-gram] radiographic images of an injected dye as it is processed and eliminated by the kidney

exercise stress test [EKS-er-zyz STRES test] a cardiac assessment that determines heart rate, blood pressure, and electrocardiography (ECG) while exercising at various intensities, usually on a treadmill

exercise-induced asthma [EKS-er-zyz-in-DOOST AZ-mah] a subtype of asthma where bronchoconstriction and dyspnea are triggered by physical exertion

exercise-induced urticaria [EKS-er-zyz-in-DOOST ur-tih-KAR-ee-uh] large, red, raised lesions of the skin resulting from histamine release during exercise

exhalation [eks-ha-LAY-shun] the process of pushing air out of the lungs

exo- [eks-oh] *prefix*; outside, external

exogenous [eks-OH-jeh-nus] originating outside an organ or body part

exophthalmos [eks-off-THAL-mohs] outward bulging of the anterior surface of the eye with a startled, staring expression; when presentation is unilateral, etiology is often a tumor behind the eye, but when presentation is bilateral, the patient usually has hyperthyroidism

exotoxin [eks-oh-TOK-sin] formation of excess bone tissue on the surface of a bone; also called an osteoma

exotropia [eks-oh-TROH-pee-ah] outward turning of the eyeball

expectorate [ek-SPEK-tor-ate] to cough up and expel mucus from the airway

expiratory reserve volume (ERV) [eks-PY-rah-tor-ee ree-ZEERV VOL-yoom] the volume of air exiting the lungs combined with tidal volume (TV) during forced exhalation; average value = 1,000 cc

exploratory laparotomy [eks-PLOR-ah-tor-ee LAP-ah-ROT-oh-mee] surgical procedure that uses an abdominal incision to open the abdominopelvic cavity for scrutiny

exstrophy [EK-stroh-fee] extrusion of a hollow organ, such as the bladder, causing it to be turned inside out due to congenital malformation

extensor muscles [eks-TEN-sur MUS-selz] muscles that extend or stretch a limb or part

extensor muscles of the hand [eks-TEN-sur MUS-selz uv the hand] collective group of muscles on the dorsal surface of the forearm that function to extend the hand and wrist; includes the extensor carpi, radialis longus, and radialis brevis muscles

external [eks-TER-nal] outside or exterior of the body or organ

external acoustic meatus [eks-TER-nal ah-KYOOS-tik mee-AY-tus] outer segment of the ear canal

external carotid artery [eks-TER-nal ka-ROT-id AR-ter-ee] a large blood vessel of the neck that carries oxygenated blood to the thyroid gland, face, throat, and mandible

external fixation [eks-TER-nal fik-SAY-shun] surgical procedure used to treat a complicated fracture using application of metal pins that are inserted in the bone on either side of the fracture and connected to a metal frame to immobilize a fracture or lengthen a congenitally short leg

external genitalia [eks-TER-nal jen-ih-TAL-ee-ah] genitalia on the outside of the body; includes the scrotum, testes, epididymis, and penis in males; and labia, clitoris, and urethra in females

external iliac artery [eks-TER-nal IL-ee-ak AR-ter-ee] the large, more superficial division of the common iliac artery that extends down into the thigh and becomes the femoral artery

external jugular vein [eks-TER-nal JUG-yoo-lar vayn] the paired, bilateral blood vessels of the neck that return blood from the head and neck to the heart

external oblique muscle [eks-TER-nal OH-bleek MUS-sel] a bilateral muscle of the lateral chest that begins at the fifth ribs and inserts into the anterior iliac crest, serving the function of compressing the abdomen and maintaining an upright posture

extracellular fluid [EKS-trah-SEL-yoo-lar FLOO-id] liquid in the body that is outside the cells

extracorporeal [eks-trah-kor-POR-ee-al] outside the body

extracorporeal circulation [eks-trah-kor-POR-ee-al sir-kyoo-LAY-shun] shunting of blood outside the body to a device that performs a body function, blood is then returned to the patient's circulatory system;

examples include the use of a heart-lung machine or kidney dialysis

extracorporeal lithotripsy [eks-trah-kor-POR-ee-al lith-oh-TRIP-see] a therapeutic procedure in which shock waves are transmitted to the kidneys to break apart renal calculi; also known as extracorporeal shock wave lithotripsy

extraocular [eks-trah-OK-yoo-lar] anatomical region immediately adjacent to or near the outside surface of the eye

extraocular muscles [eks-trah-OK-yoo-lar MUS-selz] muscles that control the movements of the eye

extrapyramidal side effects (EPS) [ECKS-trah-pih-RAM-ih-dal SIDE ee-FEKTS] an untoward effect of neuroleptic medications with distressing symptoms including tremors, bradykinesia, dystonia, and restless movements of the mouth, legs, and hands

extraurethral incontinence [EKS-trah-yoo-re-thral in-KON-tin-ens] loss of control of urine flow caused when the sphincter mechanism has been bypassed

extravasation [EKS-trav-ah-SAY-shun] damage to tissue of the vein and surrounding structures when a chemotherapeutic drug leaks into the soft tissue surrounding the infusion site

extremity [eks-TREM-ih-tee] referring to legs, arms, and phalanges

extrinsic asthma [eks-TRIN-sik AZ-mah] asthma caused by an environmental allergen

extubation [eks-too-BAY-shun] removal of a tube, especially an endotracheal tube

exudate [EKS-yoo-dayt] movement of fluid from a vessel wall into a body cavity or adjacent tissue; often occurring due to inflammatory processes

exudative [eks-YOO-day-tiv] substance that leaks into or out of tissues

F

factitious disorder [fak-TISH-us dis-OR-der] physical and/or psychological symptoms that are consciously fabricated by the patient; pretending to be sick (often with symptoms that are difficult to evaluate)

false ribs [FAHLS ribz] the five lower costal bones on either side of the chest that do not attach directly to the sternum

false vocal cords [FAHLS VOH-kal kordz] vestibular folds in the larynx that do not produce sounds

Farre's tubercles [FARZ TOO-ber-kulz] malignant masses on the surface of the liver

fascia [FASH-uh] fibrous connective tissue that covers, supports, and separate muscles

fasciculation [fah-sik-yoo-LAY-shun] uncontrollable, localized contraction of a single muscle group that is visible through the skin

fasciectomy [fash-ee-EK-toh-mee] excision of the fascia that covers the surface of a muscle

fasciorrhaphy [fash-ee-OR-ah-fee] suturing of the fascia that covers the surface of a muscle

febrile [FEE-brile] having an elevated temperature

fecal incontinence [FEE-kul in-KONT-in-ens] inability to control defecation

fecalith [FEE-kah-lith] hardened feces that become a stonelike mass, occurring most often in the appendix or a diverticulum

feces [FEE-seez] end product of digestion comprised of undigested fibers and liquid; also called stool

femoral artery [FEM-or-al AR-tur-ee] blood vessel of the medial aspect of the thigh that carries oxygenated blood; originates at the external iliac artery and terminates at the popliteal artery behind the knee

femoral vein [FEM-or-al vayn] blood vessel of the thigh that returns blood from the lower leg, starting at the popliteal vein and ending at the iliac vein

femoris anterior muscle [FEM-or-is an-TEER-ee-or MUS-sel] large muscle mass of the upper leg composed of four smaller muscles (rectus femoris, vastus lateralis, vastus medialis, and vastus intermedius), which work together to extend the leg and are often referred to simply as quadriceps

femur [FEE-mur] thighbone extending from the hip to the knee

fenestra [fe-NES-trah] small opening to relieve pressure; microscopic openings in capillaries for the purpose of filtration within the glomerular capillaries of the kidneys

ferritin [FAIR-ih-tin] blood chemistry test, used to diagnose iron deficiency anemia, that indirectly measures the amount of iron stored in the body by measuring the small amount that is always present in the blood

ferrotherapy [fer-oh-THER-ah-pee] treatment of anemia by administration of iron compounds

fertilization [fer-tih-ly-ZAY-shun] union of a sperm and egg that develops into an embryo

festination [FES-tih-nay-shun] to increase in speed or rate; commonly associated with the gait pattern of individuals with Parkinson's disease

fetal alcohol syndrome [FE-tal AL-ko-hol SIN-drom] fetal development which is impaired by maternal consumption of alcohol; commonly demonstrated in the infant by craniofacial abnormalities, limb defects, and some mental retardation

fetometry [fee-TOM-eh-tree] estimation of the size, age, and growth of a fetus using ultrasonography

fetoscope [FEE-toe-skope] a fibro-optical device used for direct visualization of an embryo; historical term for stethoscope used to listen to fetal heart sounds

fibrillation [fib-ril-LAY-shun] exceedingly rapid contractions or twitching of muscular fibrils, but not of the muscle as a whole

fibroadenoma [fye-bro-ad-eh-NOH-mah] formation of firm, densely fibrous, benign tumors in glandular tissue; frequently observed in the breast

fibromyalgia [fye-bro-migh-AL-jee-uh] widespread muscle and joint pain of unknown origin

fibromyositis [FYE-bro-mi-oh-SIGH-tis] chronic muscle inflammation with hyperplasia of the connective tissue

fibroplasia [FYE-bro-PLAY-zee-ah] overproduction of fibrous tissue

fibrosis [fye-BROH-sis] increase or abnormal growth of fibrous or connective tissue in reparative or reactive processes

fibula [FIB-yoo-lah] the anterior bone of the lower leg that extends from the knee and terminates at the lateral aspect of the ankle

-fida [fy-dah] *suffix*; split

fifth cranial nerve (CN V) [fifth KRA-nee-ahl nerv] trigeminal nerve which stimulates the face and upper neck

filiform papillae [FIL-ih-form pa-PIL-ee] condition of having numerous elongated cone-shaped keratinic projections on the dorsal surface of the tongue

filtration [fil-TRAY-shun] to strain or separate by passing liquid through a device to separate wanted from unwanted substances, as in dialysis

fimbria [FIM-bree-uh] finger- or fringe-shaped projections extending from the distal ends of the fallopian tubes

first-degree burn [FURST-de-GREE burn] damage to the epidermal layer; burned-tissue reaction as a result of thermal, radioactive, chemical, or electrical insult

fiss- [fis] *prefix*; a split or cleft

fissures [FISH-urz] cracks in the skin or other tissues

fistula [FIST-yoo-lah] abnormal passage that connects two structures

flaccid [FLAS-sid] having poor or absent muscle tone

flaccid paralysis [FLAS-sid par-RAHL-ih-sis] defective, poor, or absent muscle control caused by a nerve lesion

flagellum [fla-JEL-um] a whiplike structure that propels sperm

flail chest [FLAYL chest] condition where three or more consecutive ribs have fractured in close proximity; this creates instability of the wall of the thorax, moving opposite to the normal direction during respiratory movements

flatulence [FLAT-yoo-lens] excessive gas in the intestinal tract, in the stomach or intestines

flatus [FLAY-tus] intestinal gas that is the end product of bacteria in the large intestine feeding on undigested food

flex- [fleks] *prefix*; bend

flexion [FLECK-shun] bending movement at a joint

flexor muscles [FLEKS-or MUS-selz] muscles that bend or flex a limb or part

floaters [FLO-terz] clumps of gel or cellular debris within the vitreous; these are experienced as small specks seen moving across the visual field

floating ribs [FLO-ting ribz] the 11th and 12th ribs, which do not attach to the sternum

fluorescein angiography [floo-oh-RES-sen an-jee-OG-rah-fee] diagnostic procedure in which fluorescein, an orange fluorescent dye, is injected intravenously, traveling to the retinal artery in the eye and causing it to glow fluorescent green on flash photography of the retina

fluoroscopy [floor-OS-koh-pee] examination of deep tissues and structures of the body by x-ray using a fluoroscope

-flux [fluks] *suffix*; flow

focus charting [FO-kus CHAR-ting] documentation method using a columnar format to chart data, action, and response

Foley catheter [FOH-lee KATH-eh-ter] a urethrally inserted urine drainage tube with an inflatable retaining balloon

follicle [FOL-ih-kul] space containing the hair root

folliculitis [fol-IK-yoo-LYE-tis] inflammation of the hair follicles

fontanel [fawn-tah-NEL] non-ossified membrane covering the anterior portion of the skull of a fetus; located between the cranial bones, commonly called "the soft spot"

foramen [foh-RAY-men] an opening in a bone through which nerves, blood vessels, and other structures pass

foramen magnum [foh-RAY-men MAG-num] a large opening at the base of the cranium near the occipital bone that the spinal cord passes through as it connects with the medulla oblongata

forebrain [FOR-brayn] the anterior portion of the brain including the telencephalon and diencephalon

-form [form] *suffix*; having the manner or structure of

formication [for-mih-KAY-shun] tactile hallucination or sensation that small insects are crawling under the skin; frequently associated with alcohol detoxification

fornix [FOR-niks] a tract of myelinated nerves along the arched floor of the lateral ventricles, connecting the hippocampus in each temporal lobe to the thalamus and each amygdaloid body

fossa [FAW-sah] a shallow depression in a bone or tissue

fourth cranial nerve (CN IV) [forth KRA-nee-ahl nerv] trochlear nerve; innervates the sensory and motor function of the superior oblique muscle of the eye

fourth heart sound [forth hart sownd] sound produced by the heart during late systole due to ventricular atrial systole and decreased ventricular compliances; often associated with ventricular hypertrophy, hypertension, and myocardial infarction

fovea [FOH-vee-ah] a natural depression on a body surface such as a bone

fovea visuala [FOH-vee-ah viz-OO-ah-lah] a small depression in the center of the macula, directly opposite the pupil, where the greatest visual acuity lies

Fowler position [FOW-ler po-ZISH-un] semireclining in bed, with head of bed elevated

fracture [FRAK-chur] breakage of bone due to injury or disease process; classified according to the direction of the break or degree of disruption of structural integrity

fragile X syndrome [FRAJ-il ex SIN-drom] a disorder caused by extra genetic fragments on the X chromosome, resulting in mental retardation, distinctive facial deformity, and macro-orchidism

free radicals [free RAD-ih-kalz] atoms or groups of atoms that can cause damage to cells

fremitus [FREM-ih-tus] palpable vibration; crackles or thrill from body cavities or joints; subtypes include tactile, vocal, and tussive

frenulum [FREN-yoo-lum] an elongated connective structure that attaches two parts such as the posterior surface of the tongue and upper lip at the gum line

friction rub [FRIK-shun rub] abnormal grating sounds detected during auscultation when pleura or pericardial tissues are inflamed

frontal bone [FRON-tal bohn] large bone of the cranium that forms the forehead and superior portions of the orbits

frontal lobe [FRON-tal lohb] the portion of each cerebral hemisphere located anterior to the central sulcus

frontal sinus [FRON-tal SY-nus] a hollow space in the area of the forehead

frontalis muscle [fron-TAL-is MUS-sel] muscle that covers the frontal bone

fructosuria [FRUK-tos-YUR-ee-ah] excretion of fructose in the urine

-fuge [fyooj] *suffix*; to drive away; having a fleeting quality

fulguration [ful-gyoo-RAY-shun] destruction of unwanted tissue by the use of electrical current in the form of sparks

full thickness graft [ful THIK-nes graft] surgical transplantation of the epidermis and underlying tissues

fundus [FUN-dus] the area furthest from the opening

fungating [FUN-gayt-ing] rapid growth similar to fungus; used to describe some quick-developing tumors

furuncle [FUR-ung-kul] a boil

fusiform aneurysm [FEW-zi-form AN-yoo-riz-um] spindle-shaped protrusion on an artery

G

gag reflex [GAG REE-fleks] response by the throat that causes retching

gait apraxia [gayt ah-PRAK-see-uh] loss of the ability to consciously sequence and execute the movements required to coordinate walking, resulting in unsteady walking patterns; widely based, jerky gait, and balance difficulties as demonstrated in Parkinson's disease

galactocele [ga-LAK-tow-seel] a cyst caused by an occluded lactiferous duct in the breast

gallbladder [GALL-blad-der] a pear-shaped pouch on the inferior surface of the right hepatic lobe that stores bile

gallium [GAL-ee-um] a radioisotope utilized in diagnostic scans for neoplasm, inflammation, and soft-tissue disorders

gamete [GAM-eet] spermatozoa from the male or ova from the female; cells that have only 23 chromosomes rather than the usual 46

gamma-amino butyric acid (GABA) [GAM-ah-ah-MEE-noh byu-TER-ik AS-id] an amino acid that functions as an inhibitory neurotransmitter in the brain and spinal cord

ganglion cyst [GANG-lee-on sist] a fluid-filled mass most often observed in the wrist, but may also occur on the ankle

ganglionectomy [gang-glee-ohn-EK-tuh-mee] excision of a ganglion

ganglionic cyst [GANG-glee-ohn-ik sist] a benign cyst localized on or around a tendon sheath or joint capsule

gangrene [GANG-green] necrosis of a body tissue

gastralgia [gas-TRAL-gee-uh] pain in the stomach

gastrectomy [gas-TREK-toh-mee] surgical removal of part or all of the stomach

gastric [GAS-trik] pertaining to the stomach

gastric bypass [GAS-trik BY-pass] surgical creation of a small stomach pouch with anastomosis of the stomach with the jejunum, reducing caloric absorption as a treatment for morbid obesity

gastrinoma [gas-trin-OH-mah] a tumor associated with Zollinger-Ellison syndrome that secretes gastrin

gastritis [gas-TRY-tis] acute or chronic inflammation of the stomach due to excess acid production or a bacterial infection

gastrocele [GAS-troh-seel] herniation or protrusion of part of the stomach

gastrocnemius muscle [gas-trok-NEE-mee-us MUS-sel] muscle of the posterior surface of the lower leg that, when flexed, initiates plantar flexion

gastroenteritis [gas-troh-en-tur-EYE-tis] stomach and intestinal inflammation resulting from infection

gastroenterologist [gas-troh-en-ter-AWL-oh-jist] physician who practices in the medical specialty of gastroenterology, diagnosing and treating patients with diseases of the gastrointestinal system

gastroenterology [gas-troh-EN-ter-AWL-oh-jee] study of the stomach and intestines

gastroesophageal [gas-troh-ee-sof-ah-JEE-ul] pertaining to the esophagus and stomach

gastroesophageal reflux disease [gas-troh-ee-sof-ah-JEE-ul REE-fluks dis-EEZ] disorder of stomach contents being regurgitated into the esophagus

gastrointestinal [gas-troh-en-TES-tih-nal] pertaining to the stomach and intestines

gastroparesis [gas-troh-pah-REE-sis] reduced contractility of the stomach

gastroplasty [GAS-troh-plas-tee] surgical procedure for severe obesity in which the size and volume capacity of the stomach are reduced by staples or intestinal bypass

gastrorrhaphy [gas-TROR-ah-fee] suturing or sewing an injured stomach wall

gastroscopy [GAS-tros-skop-ee] visualization of the esophagus, stomach, and duodenum using a fiberoptic endoscope

gastrospasm [GAS-troh-spazm] sudden, involuntary, and painful contraction of the stomach muscles

gastrostomy [gas-TROWS-toh-mee] surgical creation of a permanent opening from the abdominal wall into the stomach to insert a gastrostomy tube

-gen [jen] *suffix*; production or origin

-genesis [jen-ee-sis] *suffix*; produce or originate

genital [JEN-ih-tal] pertaining to the reproductive organs of male and female

genitourinary system [JEN-ih-toh-YOO-rih-nair-ee SIS-tem] comprised of the kidney, ureters, and bladder

genotype [JEN-oh-type] the genetic makeup of an individual

genu valgum [JEEN-yoo VAL-gum] congenital deformity in which the lower legs are bent medially; also known as knock-knee

genu varum [JEEN-yoo VA-rum] congenital deformity in which the lower legs are bent away from the midline; also known as bowleg

geriatrics [jer-ee-AT-riks] branch of medicine dealing with care and treatment of problems particular to old age

germinal cell [JER-min-al sell] a tissue from which other tissues or cells proliferate

germinal centers [JER-min-al SEN-terz] areas of rapidly dividing lymphocytes within the lymph nodules that respond to infection by forming and releasing lymphocytes for combat

germinal stage [JER-min-al STAYJ] developmental stage that begins with conception and lasts approximately 10 to 14 days

gero- [jer-oh] *prefix*; elderly, old age

gerontology [jer-on-TOL-oh-jee] the study of the problems particular to old age and the aging process

gestalt therapy [ges-TALT THAIR-ah-pee] a form of psychotherapy that emphasizes treating the whole person by focusing on relationships and responses both emotional and biological

gestation [jes-TAY-shun] length of time of the development of a fetus in utero from conception to birth

gestational diabetes mellitus [jes-TAY-shun-al dye-ah-BEE-teez mel-EYE-tus] disorder of glucose metabolism that occurs during pregnancy; type III

giardiasis [jee-ar-DI-aye-sis] infection with the parasite *Giardia lamblia* which causes diarrhea, cramping, and dyspepsia

gingival hyperplasia [jin-JYH-val hy-per-PLAY-zee-uh] overgrowth of gum tissue commonly observed in patients treated with anticonvulsants

gingivitis [jin-jih-VY-tis] inflammation of the tissue (gums) immediately adjacent to the teeth

gingivoglossitis [JIN-jih-voh-glaw-SY-tis] inflammation of the gums and tongue

gland [gland] any one of many organs in the body comprised of specialized cells that secrete or excrete materials not related to their ordinary metabolism

Glasgow coma scale [GLAS-goh KOH-mah SKAYL] a clinical observation scale used to document level of consciousness

glaucoma [glaw-KOH-mah] increased intraocular pressure (IOP) because the aqueous humor cannot circulate freely; in open-angle glaucoma, the angle where the edges of the iris and cornea touch is normal and open, but the trabecular meshwork is blocked

glenoid [GLEH-noyd] resembling a socket of a joint; the depressed or indented articular surface

glenoid cavity [GLEH-noyd KAV-ih-tee] the depression in the scapula into which the head of the humerus fits

glenoid fossa [GLEH-noyd FAW-sah] a shallow depression where the head of the humerus joins the scapula to make the shoulder joint

-glia [glee-ah] *suffix*; substance that holds matter together

glioma [GLEE-oh-mah] tumor of glial cells graded by degree of invasion

global amnesia [GLOH-bal am-NEE-zee-ah] loss of all memories

glomerular filtration [gloh-MER-yoo-lur fil-TRAY-shun] the rate at which blood is filtered at the glomerulus;

clearance test used to determine the glomerular filtrating rate

glomerulonephritis [gloh-mer-yoo-loh-nef-RIGH-tis] an inflammatory disease of the kidney typically occurring one to two weeks after a streptococcal bacterial infection; symptoms include hematuria and proteinuria

glomerulosclerosis [gloh-mer-yoo-loh-skle-ROH-sis] fibrosis of the renal glomeruli

glossal [GLOS-al] relating to the tongue

glossectomy [glaw-SEK-toh-mee] surgical revision or complete excision of the tongue

glossitis [glaw-SY-tis] inflammation of the tongue which may be caused by irritation from food, infection, or vitamin B deficiency

glossorrhaphy [glos-SOR-ah-fee] application of sutures to the tongue

glottis [GLOT-tis] the vocal apparatus of the larynx, including the vocal folds, vocal chords, vocal muscles, and adjacent structures of the throat

glucagon [GLOO-kuh-gon] pancreatic hormone from alpha cells that elevates blood glucose

glucogenesis [glu-koh-JEN-eh-sis] formation of sugar from fats and proteins

glucometer [GLU-koh-mee-ter] a device used to measure blood levels of glucose

glucose tolerance test [GLU-kos TOL-er-ans test] diagnostic study in which the patient is administered 75 g of glucose while fasting, with measurement of blood glucose at regular intervals to determine ability to regulate glucose metabolism

glucosuria [GLOO-kohs-YOOR-ee-ah] presence of glucose (sugar) in the urine

gluten enteropathy [GLOO-tin en-tur-OWP-ah-thee] malabsorption and gastric irritation due to gluten sensitivity; celiac sprue, celiac disease

gluteus [GLYOO-tee-us] referring to the buttocks

gluteus maximus muscle [GLYOO-tee-us MAK-sih-mus MUS-sel] large muscle forming the buttocks that extends to the thigh

gluteus medius muscle [GLYOO-tee-us MEE-dee-us MUS-sel] middle, smaller muscle in the buttock region that extends to the thigh

glycohemoglobin [GLYE-ko-HEE-moh-glo-bin] a hemoglobin A molecule with a glucose group on the N-terminal valine amino acid unit of the beta chain

glycolysis [gly-KOL-ih-sis] energy-yielding conversion of glucose to lactic acid in the tissues

glycosylated hemoglobin [GLYE-kos-ih-lay-ted HEE-moh-gloh-ben] used to test circulating glucose blood levels over the life span of a red blood cell

gnath- [nath] *prefix*; pertaining to the jaw and/or cheek

gnathoplasty [NATH-oh-plas-tee] surgical reconstruction of the jaw

-gogue [gog] *suffix*; to make flow

goiter [GOY-tur] enlargement of the thyroid gland

goniometer [goh-nee-AWM-eh-ter] a protractor-like device used to measure the angle and degrees of range of movement (ROM) of a joint

gonioscopy [goh-nee-AWS-koh-pee] use of a slit lamp with a special lens that illuminates the trabecular meshwork

gonococcus [gon-oh-KOK-us] infectious agent in the sexually transmitted disease gonorrhea

gonorrhea [gon-oh-REE-ah] a sexually transmitted disease caused by the microorganism *Neisseria gonorrhea* causing inflammation of the urethra, endocervix, and fallopian tubes

gout [GOWT] disorder that occurs most often in men due to excessive levels of uric acid in the blood; acute attacks cause sudden, severe pain in the great toe or hands as uric acid moves from the blood into the soft tissues and forms masses of crystals with soft-tissue swellings known as tophi

gouty arthritis [GOW-tee arth-RY-tis] inflammation of joints due to formation of tophi from accumulation of uric acid crystals

gracilis muscle [GRAS-ih-lis MUS-sel] skeletal muscle that inserts near the pubis and extends to the medial tuberosity of the tibia; upon contraction it adducts the thigh and flexes the knee

graft [GRAFT] surgical procedure that uses skin, whole bone, or bone chips to repair areas of tissue damage

-gram [gram] *suffix*; record of

-graph [graf] *suffix*; instrument that records

-graphy [graf-ee] *suffix*; process of recording data

Graves disease [GRAYVZ dis-EEZ] a form of hyperthyroidism caused by excessive thyroid hormone production, resulting in enlargement of the thyroid gland and exophthalmos

-gravida [grav-id-ah] *suffix*; pregnancy

gray matter [gray MAT-er] brain and spinal-cord tissue made up primarily of unmyelinated fibers of cell bodies and dendrites of nerve cells

great saphenous vein [grayt sah-FEE-nus vayn] major blood vessel that returns blood along the medial surface of the thigh

greenstick fracture [GREEN-stik FRAK-shur] a break in bone with disruption of structure only on one side; occurs most often in children, as part of the bone is still composed of flexible cartilage

gross [GROHS] visible to the naked eye; large in size

guaiac [GWY-ak] a solution used to test for the presence of occult blood in fecal matter

gustation [gus-TAY-shun] sense of taste

Guthrie's test [GUTH-reez test] a routine screening test for phenylketonuria in newborns consisting of placing a small amount of blood on filter paper to detect the presence of excessive phenylalanine in the blood

gynecologist [gye-neh-KOL-oh-jist] a physician specializing in the study of diseases and treatment of the female genital tract

gynecomastia [GY-neh-koh-MAS-tee-ah] development of excessive mammary ducts or tissues in males due to mildly increased estrogen levels

-gynous [gin-us] *suffix*; having female characteristics

gyrus [JY-rus] a bulge or convolution on the surface of the cerebral cortex of the brain

H

H2 receptor antagonist [aitch-too ree-SEP-tor an-TAG-oh-nist] drug that blocks gastric secretions; proton or pump inhibition for the purpose of suppressing gastric acid secretion

hair cells [HAIR SELZ] epithelial cells with hairlike processes that respond to sound waves and maintain equilibrium

hair follicle [HAIR FOL-ih-kel] a saclike structure from which hair grows

hairline fracture [HAIR-lyne FRAK-shur] a very thin break line of the bone with pieces closely approximated, which is often difficult to detect on an x-ray

half-life [HAF-lyf] time required by the body to eliminate half of the blood concentration level of the original drug dose

Hallervorden-Spatz syndrome [HOL-eh-FOR-den-shpots SIN-drom] a degenerative neurological disorder found in children; characterized by parkinsonism, rigidity, and progressive dementia due to accumulation of iron pigments in the brain

hallucination [hal-loo-sih-NAY-shun] subjective perception of events and sensations for which there is no external basis

hallucinatory neuralgia [ha-LOO-sen-ah-tor-ee nyoo-RAL-jee-ah] sensation of localized pain following the cessation of an episode of severe throbbing pain

hallucinogen [huh-LOO-sih-noh-jen] a drug such as LSD or PCP that reduces perceptions of reality

hallucis flexus [HAL-yoo-sis FLEK-sus] permanent contracture of the great toe; commonly referred to as a hammertoe

hallux [HAL-uks] great toe, which is on the medial side of the foot

hallux rigidus [HAL-uks rih-JID-us] a painful condition of the great toe where the joint cartilage deteriorates at the articular surface of the metatarsal, resulting in painful ambulation and stiffening of the joint

hallux valgus [HAL-uks VAL-gus] deformity of the foot in which the great toe is angled laterally toward the other toes

halo traction [HAY-loh TRAK-shun] use of pins inserted into the cranium and attached to a circular metal ring, forming a halo and stabilizing cervical fractures

hamate [HAM-ayt] one of eight carpal bones located on the distal portion of the wrist

hamstring muscle group [HAM-string MUS-sel GRUP] a collective mass of muscles of the upper posterior leg that flex the leg; composed of biceps femoris, semitendinosus, and semimembranosus muscles

hard palate [hard PAL-ayte] the anterior bony portion of the roof of the mouth that contains the palatine vessels, nerves, and mucous glands

Hashimoto's thyroiditis [hah-shee-MOH-tohz THIGH-roid-eye-tis] autoimmune disease causing an inflamed thyroid gland

haustra [HOS-tra] pouchlike structures in the intestinal walls that expand and contract to hold varying amounts of food during digestion

Haversian canals [ha-VER-zhan kah-NALZ] nutrient system within compact bone that contains nerves, blood vessels, and lymphatic vessels

heart [HART] the hollow muscular organ responsible for acting as a pump for the circulation of blood

heart failure [hart FAIL-yer] condition in which the heart cannot pump enough blood to meet the metabolic requirement of body tissues due to myocardial infarction, ischemic heart disease, or cardiomyopathy

heart-lung machine [hart-LUNG mah-SHEEN] mechanical device that serves as artificial lungs and heart during some cardiac procedures

hebephrenia [HEB-ee-FREE-nee-ah] a trait associated with schizophrenia in which the patient demonstrates childish or silly behavior

Heimlich maneuver [HYM-lik man-OOV-er] procedure used to assist individuals with airway obstruction due to choking by grasping around the victim's waist from behind and applying a forceful push upward and inward to generate a burst of air to remove the obstruction

Helicobacter pylori [hel-ih-koh-BAK-ter py-LOR-eye] bacterium thought to be responsible for the majority of gastric ulcer diseases

hem- [heem] *prefix*; blood

hemangioma [hee-MAN-jee-OH-ma] congenital proliferation of blood vessels resulting in a mass; occurs frequently in the skin and subcutaneous tissue

hemarthrosis [HEE-mar-THROH-sis] blood in the joint cavity from blunt trauma or penetrating wound, or occurring spontaneously in hemophiliac patients

hematemesis [hem-ah-TEM-esis] vomiting of new or old blood from bleeding stomach or esophagus; can be caused by an esophageal ulcer, esophageal varix, or gastric ulcer

hematochezia [he-MAH-toh-KEE-zee-ah] blood in the stool due to an ulcer, Crohn's disease, polyp, diverticulum, or hemorrhoid

hematocrit [hee-MAT-oh-krit] a laboratory test that determines the percentage of erythrocytes in a blood sample

hematologist [HEE-mah-TAWL-oh-jist] physician who practices the medical specialty of blood disorders and blood-forming tissues

hematometra [HEE-mah-toh-ME-trah] collection of blood in the uterine cavity

hematuria [hee-muh-TUR-ee-ah] abnormal presence of blood in the urine

hemi- [hem-ee] *prefix*; one-half

hemianalgesia [HEM-ee-an-al-JEE-zee-ah] loss of sensitivity to pain on one side of the body

hemianopia [HEM-ee-ah-NOH-pee-ah] loss of vision in half of the normal visual field (right or left, top or bottom)

hemiataxia [HEM-ee-ah-TAX-ee-ah] loss of muscular control affecting one side of the body, often due to stroke or traumatic injury of the cerebellum

hemiazygos vein [HEM-ee-ah-ZY-gos vayn] one of the blood vessels of the thorax that begins in the left ascending lumbar vein, proceeds through the thorax, and eventually goes up to the azygous vein

hemicolectomy [HEM-ih-koh-LEK-toh-mee] excision of half of the colon

hemiparesis [HEM-ee-pah-REE-sis] partial paralysis; weakness on the right or left half of the body

hemiplegia [hem-ee-PLE-jee-ah] paralysis on one side of the body

hemiplegic gait [hem-ee-PLE-jik gayt] manner of walking with a stiff, extended leg, lacking any flexion of the knee or ankle, resulting in a semicircular movement of the foot with each step

hemispasm [HEM-ee-spazm] involuntary, painful muscular contractions of one side of the body or face

hemodialysis [hem-oh-dye-AL-ih-sis] filtering of blood through an external machine that stands in for the kidneys; used in cases of renal failure and some toxic conditions

hemodialyzer [hem-oh-DYE-uh-lye-zur] machine that acts as an artificial kidney during dialysis

hemodynamics [HEE-moh-dy-NAM-iks] pressures generated by blood and passage of blood through the heart and pulmonary system

hemoglobin A [HEE-moh-gloh-bin AYE] normal hemoglobin that binds with oxygen and carbon dioxide

hemolytic uremic syndrome [hem-oh-LIT-ik ur-REE-mik SIN-drom] a rare kidney disorder with onset usually in infancy that presents with renal failure, destruction of red blood cells, and platelet deficiency; treatment includes dialysis and conservative treatment with good prognosis for infants and children, but less optimistic outcomes for adults

hemophilia [HEE-moh-FIL-ee-ah] an inherited genetic abnormality of a gene on the X chromosome, causing a lack or a deficiency of a specific clotting factor; disorder causes permanent tendency toward spontaneous and traumatic episodes of hemorrhage

hemophilia A [HEE-moh-FIL-ee-ah AYE] inherited blood disorder resulting in the absence of clotting factor VIII; this is the most common type of hemophilia, occurring almost exclusively in males

hemophilia B [HEE-moh-FIL-ee-ah BEE] inherited blood disorder resulting in the absence of clotting factor IX

hemophilia C [HEE-moh-FIL-ee-ah SEE] inherited blood disorder resulting in the absence of clotting factor XI

hemoptysis [hee-MOP-ti-sis] coughing up blood or blood-tinged mucus

hemorrhagic stroke [hem-oh-RAJ-ik STROK] sudden bleeding in the brain that disrupts the supply of nutrients to the brain

hemorrhoid [HEM-or-royd] swollen, protruding veins in the rectum; usually described as being internal or external

hemosiderosis [HEE-moh-sid-er-OH-sis] increased storage of iron in body tissues; associated with diseases involving the destruction of red blood cells; for example, hemolytic anemia

hemostasis [HEE-moh-stay-sis] to stop bleeding; stabilize input and output of a system

hemostatic forceps [hee-moh-STAT-ik FORE-seps] clamping tool with a clasp that holds the blades in a closed position; used to stop blood flow at the end of a blood vessel and control hemorrhage; often called "hemostat"

hemothorax [hem-oh-THOR-aks] abnormal presence of blood in the pleural cavity

hepatatoiminodiacetic scan (HIDA) [HEP-ah-tah-toh-IM-in-oh-dy-ah-SEE-tik skan] a diagnostic imaging technique of injection of the radionuclide to obtain images of the liver, gallbladder, and biliary tree

hepatic portal [he-PAT-ik POR tul] the pathway of blood flow from the gastrointestinal (GI) tract and spleen to the liver via the portal vein and its tributaries

hepatic portal circulation [he-PAT-ik POR-tul sir-kyoo-LAY-shun] blood vessels that divert blood from digestive organs to the liver before returning through veins back up to the heart

hepatic portal vein [he-PAT-ik POR-tul vayn] blood vessel that carries blood from the liver to the inferior vena cava

hepatitis A [hep-ah-TY-tis aye] inflammation of the liver due to infection from hepatitis A virus that is most often transmitted through contact with contaminated food or water; may be transmitted between sexual partners

hepatitis B [hep-ah-TY-tis bee] inflammation of the liver due to infection with the hepatitis B virus; symptoms may be acute or chronic, and include jaundice, nausea, vomiting, and joint pain; infection may be transmitted between sexual partners and by blood-borne exposure

hepatitis C [hep-ah-TY-tis see] inflammation of the liver due to infection with a single-stranded RNA virus by way of blood or body fluids; typical presentation of persistent elevation of liver enzymes on routine lab testing; may be transmitted between sexual partners

hepatocyte [hep-AH-toh-site] cell of liver tissue

hepatoma [hep-ah-TOH-ma] neoplastic or benign tumors of the liver

hepatomegaly [HEP-ah-toh-MEG-ah-lee] palpable abdominal enlargement of the liver due to damage from cirrhosis or hepatitis

hepatosplenomegaly [HEP-ah-toh-sple-noh-MEG-ah-lee] enlargement of both the liver and the spleen

hepatotoxic [HEP-ah-toh-TOK-sik] having an overwhelmingly detrimental or destructive effect on the liver; for example, large doses of acetaminofen

hereditary disease [heh-RED-ih-tair-ee dis-EEZ] illness caused by inherited or spontaneously mutated genetic material of the cell

hernia [HUR-nee-ah] abnormal protrusion of an organ through a wall or cavity

hernia, inguinal [HUR-nee-ah, ING-gwih-nal] protrusion of abdominal structures or bowel in the groin region

hernia, reducible [HUR-nee-ah, re-DEW-si-bul] abnormal protrusion of an organ through a wall or cavity that can be physically manipulated back into normal position

herniated disc [HER-nee-ay-ted disk] protrusion of a degenerated or fragmented intervertebral disc which often causes compression of the nerve root

herniorrhaphy [her-nee-OR-ah-fee] surgical repair of an opening in the wall of a body or cavity

herpes simplex [HER-peez SIM-pleks] recurrent, painful clusters of blisters, erupting on the lips or nose and caused by infection with herpes simplex virus type 1; after the initial infection the virus is dormant in the skin until triggers of stress, sunlight, illness, or menstruation cause it to erupt again

herpes varicella [HER-peez var-ih-SELL-ah] virus that causes chickenpox

herpes zoster [HER-peez ZOS-tur] painful raised lesions along nerve roots; also called shingles

hertz [HERTS] pitch or frequency of a tone is measured in hertz (Hz)

hiatal hernia [high-AY-tul HUR-nee-ah] protrusion of the stomach and abdominal contents through the hiatal opening due to weakness in the diaphragm

Hickman catheter [HIK-man KATH-eh-ter] a central venous catheter used for administration of fluids, chemotherapy, and total parental nutrition

high-density lipoproteins [hy-DEN-sih-tee ly-poh-PRO-teenz] a fat and protein complex that removes excess cholesterol from arterial walls and transports it to the liver

hilar [HY-lar] pertaining to the indented surface of the lung

hilum [HY-lum] an indented surface of the lung; plural is hila

hindbrain [HYND-brayn] the posterior area of the brain that includes the pons and cerebellum

hippocampus [hip-oh-KAM-pus] an elongated structure with a head and a tail that is located in each temporal lobe; responsible for controlling long-term memory and facilitating comparison between present and past emotions and experiences

Hirschsprung's disease [HERSH-sproongz dis-EEZ] a congenital disorder characterized by absence of autonomic parasympathetic ganglion cells in the colon that prevents peristalsis at the diverticulum causing inadequate gastric motility and mechanical obstruction of the intestine

hirsutism [HUR-sewt-iz-um] abnormal or excessive hair growth on a female's face or body

His bundle [HIZ BUN-del] a concentration of modified cardiac fibers that conduct electronic impulses to the ventricles, ultimately dividing into the left and right bundle branches

histamine [HIS-tah-meen] a depressor amine with powerful stimulation of gastric secretions, constriction of smooth muscle, and vasodilation

histamine test [HIS-tah-meen test] a diagnostic test to determine the maximal production of gastric acidity following the administration of an antihistamine subcutaneously while gastric contents are removed by a nasogastric tube for laboratory analysis

histocyte [HISS-toh-syt] a phagocytic cell present in connective tissue; occurs naturally as part of the body's immune system

histology [his-TAWL-oh-jee] study of tissues

Hodgkin's disease [HOJ-kins dis-EEZ] malignant lymphoma with characteristic large multinucleated cells, occurring in a single lymph node of the neck, axilla, or groin, spreading to adjacent nodes and tissues if left untreated

Hofmeister operation [HAWF-my-ster op-er-AYE-shun] partial gastrectomy with suturing of the lesser curvature of the stomach and anastomosis of the jejunum

Holter monitor [hol-ter MON-ih-ter] recording of cardiac activity by a portable device which the patient wears for as long as 24 hours

Homans sign [HO-manz syn] presence of pain in the calf of the leg with dorsiflexion of the foot that is indicative of thrombophlebitis or thrombosis

homeostasis [HOH-mee-oh-STAY-sis] condition of equilibrium in which the internal state of the body is maintained by ongoing processes of feedback and regulatory functions in response to internal and external conditions

homicidal ideation [HOHM-ih-SY-dal EYE-dee-AA-shun] to have thoughts, ideas, or plans to commit murder or serious bodily harm to another person as a symptom of a psychiatric disorder or delirium

homo- [hoh-moh] *prefix*; same or alike

hordeolum [hor-DEE-oh-lum] red, painful swelling or pimple containing pus near the edge of the eyelid that is caused by a bacterial infection (*Staphylococcus*) in a sebaceous (meibomian) gland

horizontal fissure [hor-ih-ZON-tal FISH-ur] anatomical landmark of the right lung that separates the superior and middle lobes

horizontal plane [hor-ih-ZON-tal PLAYN] level to the ground

hormone [HOR-mohn] chemical messenger found in the blood

hormone-replacement therapy [HOR-mohn-ree-PLAYS-ment THER-a-pee] hormone administration to restore normal function

hospice [HOS-pis] an end-of-life, multidisciplinary treatment provided to clients experiencing the end months of life; focuses on palliation, or relief of suffering

human growth hormone (HGH) [HYOO-man grohth HOR-mohn] substance secreted by the anterior pituitary gland that regulates cellular division and protein synthesis required for normal growth of tissues

human immunodeficiency virus (HIV) [HYOO-man im-YOO-noh-de-FISH-en-see VY-rus] retrovirus that causes acquired immunodeficiency syndrome (AIDS), resulting in loss of immune function and subsequent opportunistic infections

human papilloma virus (HPV) [HYOO-man pap-il-LOH-mah VY-rus] a sexually transmitted agent that causes genital warts and severe cervical intraepithelial neoplasia; it is a precursor to cervical cancer

humerus [HYOO-mer-us] the long bone in the upper arm that articulates with the scapula at the shoulder joint and the head of the radius and ulna to form the elbow joint

humoral immunity [HUGH-mor-ul im-YOO-ni-tee] immune response maintained by antibodies; antigens stimulate the production of an antibody

Huntington's chorea [HUN-ting-tunz koh-REE-ah] a hereditary disease of the central nervous system characterized by bizarre involuntary movements and progressive dementia

hyaline membrane disease [HY-ah-lin MEM-brayn dis-EEZ] respiratory disease characterized by a collapsed alveoli due to the lack of surfactant, a substance produced by the lungs to keep the alveoli inflated

hydrarthrosis [hy-drar-THRO-sis] accumulation of serous fluid in a joint

hydro- [high-droh] *prefix*; water or fluid

hydrocele [HY-dro-seel] any accumulation of fluid around the testicle

hydrocephalus [high-dro-SEF-ah-lus] abnormal accumulation of cerebrospinal fluid in the ventricles of the brain as a result of developmental anomalies, infection, or tumor

hydrochloric acid [HIGH-droh-klor-ik AS-id] an aqueous solution of hydrogen chloride

hydrometer [HIGH-droh-mee-ter] a device used to determine the specific gravity of liquid by comparison to water

hydronephrosis [high-droh-neh-FROH-sis] dilation of the renal pelvis and calyces of one or both kidneys due to mechanical obstruction of the flow of urine by tumor, calculus, or inflammation or obstruction of the prostate or edema

hydrosalpinx [hy-droh-SAL-pinks] serous fluid in the fallopian tube

hydrosis [high-DROH-sis] sweat production and excretion

hydroxycorticosteroid [high-DROK-see-kor-ti-koh-STER-oid] analysis of urine to detect cortisol byproducts

hymen [HY-men] thin membranous folds of tissue that partially occlude the ostium of the vagina; it is sometimes absent or disrupted even without sexual activity

hyoid bone [HY-oyd bohn] a flat, U-shaped bone that does not touch any other bones but functions as a bony bridge that anchors the muscles of the tongue

hyper- [high-per] *prefix*; above, elevated

hyperaldosteronism [HY-per-al-DOS-ter-ohn-izm] excessive production of aldosterone altering the regulation of potassium and sodium exchange in the distal renal tubule

hyperalimentation [HY-per-al-ih-men-TAY-shun] enteral or parenteral infusion of a solution containing complete nutritional requirements for normal growth, development, and tissue repair

hyperbilirubinemia [hy-per-BIL-ih-roo-bih-NEE-mee-uh] an abnormally high concentration of bilirubin in the circulating blood, resulting in jaundice

hypercalcemia [high-per-kal-SEE-mee-ah] abnormally high level of calcium in the blood

hypercapnia [high-per-CAP-nee-ah] abnormally high level of carbon dioxide (CO_2) in the arterial blood

hyperemesis [high-per-EM-eh-sis] extremely severe vomiting

hyperesthesia [HIGH-per-es-THE-zee-ah] increased sensitivity to stimulation such as pressure or touch, resulting in pain

hyperextension [HIGH per-eks-TEN-shun] overstraightening; overextending beyond normal joint function or near the maximum extension

hyperglycemia [high-per-gly-SEE-mee-ah] abnormally high blood glucose level

hyperinsulinism [high-per-IN-soo-lin-izm] overproduction of insulin by the pancreas

hyperkalemia [high-per-ka-LEE-mee-ah] an abnormally high level of potassium in the blood

hyperkeratosis [HIGH-per-ker-ah-TOH-sis] overgrowth of the horny layer of the mucous membrane or epidermis

hyperkinesis [HIGH-per-kih-NEE-sis] excessive movement or activity; possible causes include hyperthyroidism or attention deficit disorder

hyperlipidemia [HIGH-per-lip-ih-DEE-mee-uh] presence of excessive amount of fats in the blood that may eventually lead to atherosclerosis

hypermetropia [high-per-meh-TROH-pee-uh] farsightedness; an error of refraction in which faraway objects appear more focused and clear than near objects

hypernatremia [high-per-nah-TREE-mee-ah] excessive level of sodium ions in the blood

hyperopia [HIGH-per-OH-pee-ah] farsightedness; inability to see objects in near visual fields clearly

hyperparathyroidism [high-per-pair-uh-THIGH-roid-izm] increased activity of parathyroid glands causing excessive parathyroid hormone (PTH) production

hyperpnea [high-purp-NEE-uh] increased depth and rate of respirations

hyperresonance [high-per-REZ-oh-nants] loud, very low-pitched, booming sounds usually heard over superinflated lungs

hypersensitivity [HIGH-per-sen-si-TIV-ih-tee] abnormal sensitivity to an allergen

hypertension [high-pur-TEN-shun] elevated blood pressure on a consistent basis with potential to cause damage to the blood vessels

hyperthyroidism [high-pur-THIGH-roid-iz-um] disorder of thyroid gland characterized by excessive thyroid hormone production

hypertonic fluid [high-per-TAWN-ik FLOO-id] liquid that is more concentrated than normal body fluid; for example, concentrated fluids used to administer some medications

hypertrichosis [high-pur-tri-KOH-sis] excessive growth of hair

hypertrophy [hy-PER-troh-fee] increase in size

hyperuricemia [high-pur-yoo-ri-SEE-mee-ah] elevated uric acid levels in the blood which cause nausea, anorexia, pruritus, and uremic frost

hyperventilation [high-pur-ven-ti-LAY-shun] increased or rapid respiratory rate that produces low alveolar carbon dioxide levels

hyphema [high-FEE-mah] blood in the anterior chamber of the eye, caused by trauma or increased intraocular pressure; treatment includes corticosteroid eyedrops or oral drugs

hypo- [high-poh] *prefix*; below, deficient or depressed

hypoalbuminemia [high-poh-al-bew-min-EE-mee-ah] abnormally low blood concentration of the protein albumin

hypoaldosteronuria [high-poh-ahl-DAWS-ter-ohn-YUR-ee-ah] abnormally low amounts of albumin in the urine

hypochondriac [high-poh-KON-dree-ak] region posterior to ribs (adjective); an individual who demonstrates morbid concern for his/her health despite absence of disease (noun)

hypochondriasis [HIGH-poh-con-DRY-ah-sis] preoccupation with bodily sensations by a patient with fear of serious illness despite medical evidence and reassurance that she/he is not ill

hypochromic [high-poh-KROH-mik] containing a lower amount of pigmentation than is normal for the bodily tissue

hypodermis [high-poh-DER-mis] innermost skin layer

hypogastric [high-poh-GAS-trik] pertaining to the area below the stomach

hypoglycemia [high-poh-gly-SEE-mee-ah] abnormally low level of blood glucose due to either inadequate caloric intake or excess insulin production

hypokalemia [HIGH-poh-kah-LEE-mee-ah] abnormally low quantity of potassium ions in circulating blood

hypokinetic dysarthria [HIGH-poh-kih-NET-ik dis-AR-three-ah] a speech disorder characterized by difficulty with regard to pitch, volume, and expressive intonation due to disorders of the extrapyramidal motor system, such as Parkinson's disease

hyponatremia [high-poh-nah-TRE-mee-ah] an abnormally low level of sodium ions in the blood

hyponychium [high-poh-NIK-ee-um] free edge portion of the nail growing beyond the phalanx tips

hypoparathyroidism [high-poh-pair-ah-THIGH-rod-izm] inadequate secretion of parathyroid hormones

hypophysis [high-POF-ih-sis] master gland that orchestrates endocrine function of the pituitary gland

hypopituitarism [high-poh-pih-TOO-eh-tar-izm] reduced or inadequate function due to pathology of the pituitary gland

hypoplasia [high-poh-PLAYZ-ee-ah] underdevelopment of an organ or tissue, often due to a decrease in the number of cells due to atrophy or destruction of tissue rather than the general size of an organ

hyposecretion [high-poh-seh-KREE-shun] decreased production of a substance below normal function or systemic need

hypospadias [high-poh-SPAY-dee-us] congenital defect in which the urethral opening is located on the penis ventral surface in males or within the vagina in females

hypothalamus [high-poh-THAL-ah-mus] brain structure located inferior to the thalamus that regulates temperature, appetite, thirst, sleep, behavioral patterns, and secretions from the pituitary gland

hypothermia [high-poh-THER-mee-ah] reduced body temperature, significantly below 98.6°F

hypotonic fluid [high-poh-TAWN-ik FLOO-id] liquid that is more dilute than normal body fluid; for example, hypotonic saline solution

hypoventilation [high-poh-ven-tih-LAY-shun] reduced or slowed respiratory rate that produces high alveolar carbon dioxide levels

hypovolemic shock [high-poh-voh-LEE-mik shok] condition where the circulating blood volume is sufficiently reduced such that blood pressure is insufficient to maintain tissue perfusion

hypoxia [high-POK-see-ah] oxygen deprivation to the tissues; if not resolved, this progresses to anoxia

hysterectomy [his-ter-EK-toh-mee] surgical removal of the uterus

hysterorrhaphy [his-ter-OR-ah-fee] suturing of the uterus

I

-ia [ee-ah] *suffix*; condition of

-iasis [eye-ah-sis] *suffix*; process or state of

-iatrics [ee-at-triks] *suffix*; treatment

iatrogenic [eye-AT-roh-JEN-ik] condition arising out of a treatment or procedure performed on a patient

-iatry [eye-ah-tree] *suffix*; medical treatment area or specialty

-ic [ik] *suffix*; pertaining to

-ical [ih-kal] *suffix*; pertaining to

-icle [ih-kl] *suffix*; small

icterus [IK-tar-us] yellow coloration of the conjunctivae which makes the sclerae also appear yellow

idiopathic [ID-ee-oh-PATH-ik] having no identifiable cause

idiopathic thrombocytopenic purpura [ID-ee-oh-PATH-ik THROM-boh-SY-toh-PEE-nik PUR-pyoo-rah] extensive bleeding into the skin and organs due to excessive destruction of platelets in the spleen because of autoimmune dysfunction; condition may be mild and transient in children and more recurrent and severe in adults

ileal [IL-ee-al] pertaining to the ileum

ileotomy [il-ee-OT-oh-mee] surgical excision of part or all of the ileum

ileum [IL-ee-um] a section of the small bowel responsible for the completion of digestion and absorption of food, following the jejunum, terminating in the lumen

ileus [IL-ee-us] gross absence of contractions in the small intestine following trauma, surgery, or intestinal obstruction

iliac [IL-ee-ak] pertaining to the hip bone

iliac crest [IL-ee-ak KREST] the most superior of the hip bones, distinguished by a broad, flaring rim

iliopsoas muscle [IL-ee-oh-SOH-as MUS-sel] a compound muscle comprised of the iliacus and psoas major muscles that flex the thigh

iliotibial band syndrome [IL-ee-oh-TIB-ee-al band SIN-drom] knee pain caused by mechanical friction of the iliotibial band across the lateral femoral epicondyle

ilium [IL-ee-um] the broad, splaying portion of the hip bone which joins the pubis and the ischium, forming the acetabulum

immunization [im-myoo-nih-ZAY-shun] a preventative measure to boost immunity of susceptible individuals by administering killed organisms or inactivated toxins

immunoablation [im-YOO-noe-ah-BLAY-shun] systematic and deliberate destruction of a patient's immune function, usually to prepare for organ transplantation or to treat severe autoimmune disorders

immunocompromised [IM-yoo-noh-COM-proh-myzd] the state of having a deficient immune response either due to a primary immune disorder or to administration of immunosuppressive agents

immunoglobulins [im-yoo-noh-GLOB-yoo-linz] glycoproteins produced by white blood cells that function as antibodies

immunologist [im-yoo-NAWL-oh-jist] one who practices the medical specialty of immunology; who diagnoses and treats patients who have autoimmune diseases, immunodeficiency diseases, cancer, or are undergoing transplantation of organs, bone marrow, or stem cells

impedance [im-PEE-dans] resistance of the bones of the inner ear to being set into motion as a result of sound waves

imperforate anus [im-PER-for-rate AYE-nus] an abnormality present at birth in which the rectum is closed, requiring immediate surgery to allow for elimination

impetigo [im-peh-TYE-goh] contagious skin condition caused by streptococci or staphylococci bacteria

implanted cardioverter defibrillator [IM-plant-id kar-dee-oh-VER-ter dee-FIB-rih-lay-tor] a surgically implanted medical device for patients with life-threatening heart arrhythmias

impotence [IM-poh-tens] inability to achieve or maintain an erection

in situ [in SIGH-too] in a contained or localized position; not extending beyond the point of origin

inactivated vaccines [in-AK-tiv-ayt-ed vak-SEENZ] a solution that has an infective agent that has been killed or substantially weakened and does not produce disease

incentive spirometry [in-SEN-tiv spy-ROM-eh-tree] a medical device used to encourage a patient to inhale and sustain inspiratory volume to exercise lungs and prevent pulmonary complications

incision and drainage [in-SIZH-un and DRAYN-ij] surgical procedure of cutting into tissue to drain fluid

incisional biopsy [in-SIZH-un-al BY-op-see] surgical removal of a small segment of the suspect lesion for microscopic examination

incisional hernia [in-SIZH-un-al HUR-nee-ah] protrusion of the bowel or abdominal structures occurring along the suture line of a prior surgical incision

incontinent [in-CON-tin-ent] inability to voluntarily control bowel movements or bladder function

indigestion [IN-dye-JEST-jun] discomfort of the gastrointestinal (GI) tract including heartburn, acid regurgitation, pain, nausea, and vomiting

inductothermy [in-DUK-toh-ther-mee] use of electromagnetic induction to artificially produce a fever in order to treat a primary pathology

induration [IN-du-ray-shun] an area of hardened tissue, caused by various pathological states

infantile hypothyroidism [IN-fan-tile high-poh-THIGH-roid-iz-um] congenital form of hypothyroidism, formally called cretinism

infectious [in FEK shus] caused by a pathogen such as virus or bacteria

inferior [in-FEER-ee-or] beneath or lower; as in reference to structures

inferior mesenteric artery [in-FEER-ee-or mes-en-TER-ik AR ter ee] major blood supply of the intestine

inferior oblique muscle [in-FEER-ee-or ob-LEEK MUS-sel] muscle that turns the eye downward and toward the midline of the visual field

inferior rectus muscle [in-FEER-ee-or RECK-tus MUS-sel] muscle that turns the eye downward

inferior vena cava [in-FEER-ee-or VEE-nah KAY-vah] large blood vessel that receives blood from the lower limbs and the pelvic and abdominal organs; structure begins at the fifth lumbar vertebra and continues anterior to the right atrium of the heart

infiltration [in-fil-TRAY-shun] substance being infused or passing into tissue or organ(s)

inflammation [in-flam-MAY-shun] the protective response of body tissues to irritation or injury

inflammatory bowel disease (IBD) [in-FLAM-ah-tor-ee BOW-el dis-EEZ] chronic inflammation of various parts of the small and large intestines; the cause is not known; symptoms include diarrhea, bloody stools, abdominal cramps, and fever

infra- [in-frah] *prefix*; under, below, or beneath

infraspinatus bursa [in-frah-spy-NAY-tus BUR-sah] a sheath located between the tendon of the infraspinatus muscle and the capsule of the shoulder joint

infraspinatus muscle [in-frah-spy-NAY-tus MUS-sel] skeletal muscle of the upper back that originates at the infraspinous fossa of the scapula and inserts at the upper edge of the humerus; when contracted, it extends and rotates the arm laterally

inguinal [IN-gwih-nal] pertaining to the groin

inguinal lymph nodes [IN-gwih-nal lymf nohdz] lymphoid tissue located in the groin area

inguinodynia [IN-gwi-noh-DYN-ee-uh] pain in the groin area due to trauma, space-occupying tumors, or infection

inhalation [in-ha-LAY-shun] the process of drawing air into the lungs

inspection [in-SPEK-shun] visual observation of external surfaces or internal body cavities

inspiratory reserve volume (IRV) [in-SPY-ra-tory ree-ZERV VOL-yoom] the volume of air entering the lungs combined with the tidal volume (TV) during forced inhalation; average value = 3,000 cc

insulin resistance [IN-soo-lin reh-ZIS-tans] defective use of the insulin that is produced

insulin shock [IN-soo-lin shok] severe hypoglycemia produced by excess insulin and inadequate food intake; characterized by diaphoresis, tremors, restlessness, confusion, diplopia, delirium, convulsions, and circulatory collapse

integument [in-TEG-yoo-ment] the skin; comprised of all layers: the epidermis, dermis, and corium

inter- [in-ter] *prefix*; between

intercostal [in-tur-KOS-tul] muscle group that contracts and relaxes the rib cage during respiration

intercostal retractions [IN-tur-KOS-tul re-TRAK-shunz] inward movement of the soft tissue between the ribs during inspiration

intercostals [in-tur-KOS-tul] pertaining to muscles in spaces between the ribs

interferons (IFNs) [in-ter-FEER-onz] antimicrobial glycoproteins produced in response to viral invasion; their presence stimulates cytotoxic T-cell activity and amplifies macrophage action

interleukin [in-ter-LOO-kin] collective group of multifunctional cytokines; synthesized by lymphocytes, monocytes, and macrophages

intermittent claudication [in-ter-MIT-ent KLAW-di-KAY-shun] condition caused by inadequate oxygen supply to the muscles; characterized by calf muscle pain and weakness triggered by walking

internal genitalia [in-TER-nal JEN-ih-TAL-ee-ah] sexual and reproductive organs anatomically located inside the body, including the prostate in males and the ovaries, fallopian tubes, cervix, and vagina in females

internal jugular vein [in-TER-nal JUG-yoo-lar vayn] the paired, bilaterally placed blood vessels of the interior neck that receive blood from the brain and superficial structures of the neck and face

interstitial [in-ter-STISH-al] pertaining to spaces within tissue, between cells or organs; also known as intercellular

interstitial cystitis [in-ter-STISH-al sis-TYE-tis] a chronic bladder condition in which the connective tissue is inflamed; related to autoimmune or allergic responses

interstitial fluid [in-ter-STISH-al FLOO-id] the portion of the extracellular fluid that is between the cells and outside the blood and lymphatic vessels

interstitial nephritis [in-ter-STISH-al nef-RYE-tis] acute or chronic inflammation of the renal intercellular tissue and tubules, possibly due to allergic response to Sulfamide or methicillin

intervertebral disc [in-tur-VUR-te-brul disk] fibrous tissue also known as the anulus fibrosus that surrounds the gelatinous center, called the nucleus pulposus, between the adjacent vertebrae

intervertebral foramen [in-tur-VUR-te-brul for-AYE-men] the large opening between the neural arch and the body of the vertebra that accommodates the spinal cord

intima [IN-tih-muh] inner layer; tunica interns

intra- [in-trah] *prefix*; within

intra-articular fracture [IN-tra-ar-TIK-yoo-lar FRAK-chur] breakage of bone in a fashion that extends through the cartilaginous covering of the bone into the joint space

intracavitary therapy [in-trah-KAV-ih-tar-ee THER-ah-pee] radiotherapy in which one or more radioactive sources are placed within a body cavity to irradiate the walls of the body cavity or proximal tissue

intracorpreal lithotripsy [IN-trah-kor-pree-al LITH-oh-trip-see] a surgical procedure that destroys bladder stones using a flexible scope that emits electrical charges.

intracranial pressure [in-trah-KRAY-nee-al PRESH-sur] force exerted by brain tissue, cerebrospinal fluid, and blood within the cranial vault

intractable seizure [in-TRAK-tah-bul SEE-zur] seizures that are ongoing even with optimal medical management

intradermal skin test [in-trah-DUR-mul SKIN test] assessment of sensitivity to an antigen injected into the skin

intranasal [in-trah-NAY-zal] pertaining to the inside of the nose

intraocular pressure [IN-tra-OK-yoo-lar PRESH-sur] measurement of the force exerted within the eye by the intraocular fluid

intravenous (IV) [in-trah-VEE-nus] pertaining to the inside of a vein, as of a thrombus, injection, infusion, or catheter

intravenous pyelogram [in-trah-VEE-nus PIE-lo-gram] radiograph of the urinary tract to examine the structure and function of the renal calyces, renal pelvis, ureters, and urinary bladder using the intravenous injection of a radiopaque contrast medium

intravesical chemotherapy [IN-trah-VES-eh-kal KEE-moh-THER-ah-pee] instillation of chemotherapy drugs into the bladder for the purpose of killing rapidly dividing cancer cells in the bladder or kidney

intrinsic asthma [in-TRIN-sick AZ-muh] asthma of unknown cause

intro- [in-troh] *prefix*; into or within

intussusception [in-tus-suh-SEP-shun] telescoping of one segment of intestine into the lumen of an adjacent segment

inversion [in-VER-zhun] turning a body part inward

ipsi- [ip-see] *prefix*; same; like self

iris [EYE-ris] a circular tissue of the eye whose color is genetically determined

irritable bowel syndrome (IBS) [IR-rit-ah-bul BOW-el SIN-drom] a disorder that consists of severe spasms of cramping abdominal pain, diarrhea, bloating alternating with constipation, and excessive secretion of mucus from the colon; also known as spastic colon or raucous colitis

ischemia [is-KEE-mee-ah] insufficient supply of blood to tissue caused by arterial blockage

ischemic stroke [is-KEE-mik strok] diminished blood supply to a particular area due to an embolism or thrombosis

islets of Langerhans [EYE-lets uv LAHNG-er-hanz] insulin-producing cells of the pancreas

-ism [izm] *suffix*; condition

iso- [eye-soh] *prefix*; same, equal

isometric contraction [eye-soh-MET-rik kon-TRAK-shun] development of muscle tension with equal opposi-tional force

isotonic fluid [eye-soh-TAWN-ik FLOO-id] liquid that has the same concentration as normal body fluid

-ist [ist] *suffix*; person or category of agent

isthmus [IS-mus] narrow passage between two connecting body cavities or parts

-ite [ite] *suffix*; having the nature or characteristic of

-itis [eye-tis] *suffix*; inflammation

-ity [ih-tee] *suffix*; condition or state of excess

-ium [ee-um] *suffix*; tissue or structure

-ize [eyze] *suffix*; subject to

J

jaundice [JAWN-dis] yellow appearance of skin and sclera due to excess bilirubin

jejunostomy [JEH-joo-NOS-toh-mee] surgical insertion of a permanent feeding tube through the abdominal wall into the jejunum

jejunum [jeh-JOO-num] an 8-foot-long section of the small intestine

joint [JOYNT] an area where two bones come together; categorized into three types: suture, vertebral, and synovial

joint capsule [joynt CAP-sool] a fibrous layer that encases the entire joint

juxta- [juks tah] *prefix*; near, close proximity

juxtaglomerular [juks-tah-gloh-MER-yoo-lur] smooth-muscle cells found near the afferent and efferent arterioles adjacent to the glomerulus

K

Kaposi sarcoma [KAH-poh-zee sar-KOH mah] purplish-brown vascular malignancy first observed on the skin and mucous membranes, although it may become systemic; often associated with acquired immunodeficiency syndrome (AIDS)

keloid [KEE loyd] elevated, firm hyperplasia with ill-defined borders; scar site

kera- [ker-ah] *prefix*; pertaining to the cornea or to a horny substance of the skin

keratin [KAIR-ah-tin] protein associated with hair and nails; oily secretion pertaining to hair follicles and sebaceous glands

keratinization [kair-ah-tin-ih-ZAY-shun] formation of a hard crust on the skin, often with a horny shape

keratomileusis [kair-ah-toh-my-LOO-sis] surgical correction of a refractive error by reshaping the deep layer of the cornea

keratomycosis [KAIR-ah-toh-my-KOH-sis] fungal infection of the cornea

ketonuria [kee-toh-NU-ree-uh] presence of excessive amounts of ketone bodies occurring as a result of uncontrolled metabolic conditions such as diabetes mellitus or starvation

kidney [KID-nee] one of two large, bean-shaped organs located in the flank region of the back that are responsible for filtering waste products out of the blood and for formation of urine

-kine [keen] *suffix;* movement

kinesiology [kih-nee-see-OL-oh-jee] study of the muscles and body movement

kinesis [kin-EE-sis] state of movement

koilonychia [koy-loh-NIK-ee-ah] deformation of the nail bed with thin, concave edges; often associated with iron deficient anemia; also called "spooning of the nails"

Korsakoff syndrome [kor-seh-KOF SIN-drom] brain damage due to nutritional deficits associated with chronic alcoholism; characterized by severe impairment of short-term memory; patient often resorts to confabulation to compensate for gaps in memory function

Kussmaul respirations [KOOS-mawl res-pih-RAY-shunz] air hunger; rapid and deep respirations without pause

kwashiorkor [kwah-shee-OR-kor] malnutrition in children caused by inadequate intake of calories and protein

kypho- [ky-foh] *prefix;* having a curvature or hump

kyphoscoliosis [KY-foh-SKOH-lee-OH-sis] a complex abnormal curvature of the spine with components of both kyphosis and scoliosis; often treated with a back brace or surgery to fuse and straighten the spine

kyphosis [ky-FOH-sis] abnormal and excessive posterior curvature of the thoracic spine; also known as humpback or hunchback

kyphotic pelvis [ky-FAWT-ik PEL-vis] abnormal backward curvature of the lumbar spine resulting in a narrowed pelvic diameter

L

labial [LAY-bee-al] pertaining to the lips of the vagina or face

labyrinthitis [lab-rin-THY-tis] viral or bacterial infection of the semicircular canals of the inner ear, causing severe vertigo

laceration [LAS-er-AYE-shun] a deep, penetrating wound with clean borders of skin

lacrimal bones [LAK-rih-mal BONZ] small, flat bones within the eye sockets, near the lacrimal tear glands

lacrimal sac [LAK-rih-mal SAK] the upper section of the nasolacrimal duct that collects tears and other fluids

lactase [LAK-tase] enzyme excreted by the villi within the small intestine to break down the sugar lactose found in milk

lactation [lak-TAY-shun] production of milk by the breasts following pregnancy

lactation amenorrhea [lak-TAY-shun ah-men-oh-REE-ah] suppression of menses while nursing

lacteals [LAK-tee-alz] lymphatic capillaries in the small intestine that absorb and transport fatty acids and other fat soluble substances through the lymphatic system

lactic dehydrogenase test [LAK-tik dee-HIGH-droh-jen-ace test] a laboratory blood test to determine the quantity of enzymes related to muscle destruction

lactogenesis [lack-toh-JEN-ih-sis] production and secretion of milk from the breast

lactose [LAK-tohs] a disaccharide found in milk of all mammals; it is made up of the monosaccharides glucose and galactose

-lalia [lay-lee-ah] *suffix*; condition of speech

laparoscope [LAP-ar-oh-skope] use of a fiberoptic surgical device to view the inside of the body through a small incision

large intestine [larj in-TES-tin] large bowel, located between small intestine and anal opening, comprised of the cecum, appendix, colon, rectum, and anus

laryngeal [lar-IN-jee-al] pertaining to the area of the larynx

laryngectomy [lar-in-JEK-toh-mee] surgical removal of the larynx, often due to throat cancer

laryngitis [lar-in-JIGH-tis] inflammation and hoarseness of vocal cords, often due to overuse or infection

laryngoscope [lar-ING-goh-skope] an instrument used to visualize the larynx

laryngotracheotomy [LAIR-in-goh-tra-kee-OT-oh-mee] surgical removal of the larynx and upper tracheal rings, often due to advanced malignancy

larynx [LAR-inks] region of the throat starting at the base of the tongue and ending at the upper trachea encircled by nine musculocartilaginous rings

laser photocoagulation [LAY-zer foh-toh-koh-AG-yoo-LAY-shun] use of a laser to seal the retina to the tissue of the interior eye

laser thermal keratoplasty [LAY-zer THER-mal KER-ah-toh-plas-tee] treatment of refractive errors of the eye by heating the cornea to shrink the collagen fibers, reshape the eye, and change the angle of the cornea in relation to the focal point

laser-assisted in situ keratomileusis (LASIK) [LAY-zer-ah-SIS-ted in SIGH-too kair-ah-toh-my-LOO-sis] a refractive procedure to correct myopia, hyperopia, and astigmatism by creating a flap of the cornea, followed by excimer laser ablation of cornea and then replacement of the flap

lateral [LAT-er-al] pertaining to the side

lateral rectus muscle [LAT-er-al REK-tus MUS-sel] muscle that turns the eye away from the midline of the visual field

latissimus dorsi muscle [lah-TIS-ih-mus DOR-sigh MUS-sel] muscle that extends and abducts the upper arm

lavage [la-VAJ] washing out of a hollow organ using a flow of liquid

left atrium [left AYE-tree-um] the left upper chamber of the heart that receives oxygenated blood from the pulmonary veins

left lung [left lung] structure of respiration located in the left chest, comprised of the superior, middle, and inferior lobes

left pulmonary arteries [left PUL-mo-nair-ee AR-ter-eez] vessels that transport blood from the heart to the lungs

left pulmonary veins [left PUL-mo-nair-ee vaynz] vessels transporting blood from the lungs to the heart

left ventricle [left VEN-trik-ul] the left lower chamber of the heart that receives blood from the left atrium and pumps it out to the body through the aorta

Legionnaire's disease [lee-jen-AIRS dis-EEZ] a severe bacterial infection with early presentation of fever and body aches; it progresses to liver and kidney damage and possibly death

lens [LENZ] the crystalline structure of the eye

-lepsy [lep-see] *suffix*; seizure

lesion [LEE-zhun] structural or functional alterations

leukocyte [LOO-koh-sight] white blood cells including the five subtypes: lymphocytes, monocytes, neutrophils, basophils, and eosinophils; normal blood values range from 5,000 to 10,000 per cubic millimeter

leukocytosis [loo-koh-sy-TOH-sis] increase in the actual number of leukocytes in the blood

leukoderma [loo-koh-DUR-mah] loss of melanin as a result of disease

leukoplakia [loo-koh-PLAY-kee-ah] whitening of the epithelium

levator ani [le-VAY-tar AY-nigh] a muscle of the pelvic floor that supports the pelvic organs

levo- [lee-voh] *prefix;* left

levoscoliosis [LEE-voh-SKOH-lee-OH-sis] spinal curves toward the patient's left

Lewy body dementia [LU-ee BOD-ee dee-MEN-sha] cognitive deterioration with rapid decline, delusions, and agitation

ligament [LIG-ah-ment] strong, fibrous bands of connective tissue that function to hold the two bone ends to a muscle or organ

limbic lobe [LIM-bik lohb] an area of the brain located around the medial aspect of the cerebral hemispheres and superior to the corpus callosum that joins the hemispheres; also known as the cingulate gyrus

limbus [LIM-bus] transitional area of cornea where the cornea is overlapped by the sclera

lingual [LIN-gwal] adjective form referring to the tongue

lingual tonsils [LIN-gwal TAWN-silz] lymphatic tissue located on both sides of the base of the tongue in the hypopharynx

lipase [LYE-pase] digestive enzyme produced by the pancreas to emulsify fat globules in the duodenum

lipocytes [LIP-oh-sights] fat cells

lipoma [lye-POH-mah] benign, fatty tumor

-lith [lith] *suffix;* stone

-lithesis [lith-ee-sis] *suffix*; slipping

lithogenesis [LITH-oh-JEN-eh-sis] formation of a stone in the body

lithotripsy [lith-oh-TRIP-see] procedure to remove an embedded kidney stone through a percutaneous incision

lithotriptor [LITH-oh-trip-tor] instrument that generates sound waves to break up a stone in the body

liver [LIV-er] the largest solid organ of the body, located in the upper right abdominal area, that contains four lobes and is responsible for metabolic, excretory, and detoxification functions

localized [LOH-kal-eyzd] limited to a specific region or body part

-logist [loh-jist] *suffix*; specialist in study or treatment of a clinical area

-logy [loh-jee] *suffix*; study of

long QT syndrome [LONG kyoo-tee SIN-drom] a genetically transmitted rhythm disturbance that places children at risk for ventricular fibrillation and sudden death

loop of Henle [LOOP uv HEN-lee] a U-shaped segment of the renal tubule, comprised of the thin descending limb and thick ascending limb

lordosis [lor-DOH-sis] abnormal, excessive, anterior curvature of the lumbar spine; also known as swayback or lordotic curvature

lumbar [LUM-bar] pertaining to the area of the lower back between the ribs and pelvis

lumbar puncture [LUM-bar PUNK-chur] diagnostic procedure that entails removal of cerebral spinal fluid from the subarachnoid space

lumbar spine [LUM-bar spyn] the five spinal vertebrae of the lower back

lumbosacral plexus [lum-boh-SAY-krul PLECK-sus] spinal nerve network of the lumbar and sacral regions

lumen [LEW-men] space inside the tubular artery, or tube; a standardized unit of light measurement called international candles; plural is lumina

lunate [loo-NAYT] a crescent-shaped bone located in the proximal row of the carpus

lungs [LUNGZ] two bilateral, spongy, cone-shaped structures of respiration contained in the pleural cavity of the thorax

lunula [LOO-new-lah] white, semilunar area of nail near the root

luteinizing hormone [LOO-tee-ih-ny-zing HOR-mone] a hormone that stimulates interstitial cells of the testes and the corpus luteum in the ovary

Lyme disease [LIME dis-EEZ] arthritis caused by the bite of an infected deer tick; symptoms include a nonpruritic erythemic rash that expands outward, bull's-eye rash, joint pain, fever, chills, and fatigue

lymph [LIMF] fluid in the lymphatic vessels

lymph nodes [LIMF nohdz] small, kidney-shaped organs that contain large numbers of lymphocytes and macrophages; these nodes occur alone and in chains along the lymphatic duct

lymph nodules [LIMF NOD-yoolz] areas of lymphocyte formation within the lymph nodes

lymphadenopathy [lim-fad-eh-NOP-ah-thee] enlargement of the lymph nodes due to activation and proliferation of lymphocytes and phagocytes that is most often associated with infection or invasion of a lymph node by a tumor

lymphadenosis [lim-FAD-eh-NOH-sis] enlargement of the lymph nodes

lymphangioma [lim-FAN-jee-oh-ma] tumor made up of lymph vessels

lymphangioplasty [lim-FAN-jee-oh-plas-tee] establishment of artificial lymph ducts to bypass areas of blocked lymphatic circulation

lymphangitis [lim-fan-JIGH-tis] inflammation of the lymph vessels

lymphatic ducts [lim-FAH-tik dukts] channels that collect lymph from organs and regions of the body

lymphatic system [lim-FAH-tik SIS-tem] comprised of the main lymphatic duct, draining lymph from the upper right body quadrant and returning it to the bloodstream via the right subclavian vein

lymphatic vessels [lim-FAH-tik VES-selz] the efferent passage for lymph

lymphatics [lim-FAH-tiks] a vascular channel that transports lymph; singular is sometimes used as an adjective to describe the quality of being sluggish

lymphocytes [LIM-foh-sights] leukocytes (white blood cells) found in lymphatic tissue

lymphogranuloma venereum [LIM-foh-gran-yoo-LOH-mah ven-eh-REE-um] a sexually transmitted disease caused by the *Chlamydia* species that causes reddened, painless erosions of the genitals and rectum, followed by lymph node enlargement and fistulous tracts, obstructions, and infection of the perirectal lymph nodes

lymphography [lim-FOG-raf-ee] a diagnostic study in which an isotope (radioactive substance) is injected into the patient's blood, taken up by the lymphatic system, and visualized through radiographic pictures

lymphokinesis [LIM-foh-kin-EE-sis] circulation of lymph through the lymphatic vessels and lymph nodes

lymphokinetic [LIM-foh-ki-NET-ick] factors or body actions that contribute to lymph circulation; includes actions such as arterial pulses, passive compression of soft body tissues, postural changes, and skeletal muscle contractions

lymphoma [lim-FOH-mah] neoplasm of lymph tissue; also called malignant lymphoma

lyo- [ly-oh] *prefix*; loosen or dissolve

-lysis [ly-sis] *suffix*; to loosen, dissolve, or relieve

-lyte [light] *suffix*; dissolved substance

M

macro- [mak-roh] *prefix*; large or elongated

macrophage [MAK-roh-fayj] monocyte cells that have migrated from circulation into tissues and are responsible for immune response by engulfing and ingesting foreign antigens

macula lutea [MAK-yoo-lah loo-TEE-ah] a yellow-colored spot visible on the retina near the optic nerve of the retina that contains the fovea centralis, which is the point of greatest visual focus

macular degeneration [MAK-yoo-lar dee-jen-er-AY-shun] loss of central vision due to disruption of the integrity of the retina

macule [MAK-yool] small, circumscribed, discolored skin lesion

magnetic resonance imaging [mag-NET-ik REZ-oh-nans IM-aj-ing] diagnostic imaging by use of electromagnetic radiation to visualize soft tissues of the body

mal- [mal] *prefix*; bad or inadequate

malabsorption syndrome [mal-ab-SORP-shun SIN-drom] inadequate uptake of nutrients from the digestive tract that may be associated with gastrectomy, gastric bypass, or deficiency of pancrease or lactase enzymes

-malacia [mah-lay-sha] *suffix*; condition of softening

malaise [mah-LAZE] feeling unwell, often the first sign of illness

malalignment [MAL-ah-LINE-ment] arrangement of bone fragments after a fracture such that they do not heal properly

malaria [mah-LAH-ree-ah] a febrile illness with malaise, headache, fatigue, and muscular aches due to infection by protozoa from the genus *Plasmodium*

malignant [mah-LIG-nant] cancer, carcinoma, endangering health or life

malingering [mah-LING-ger-ing] demonstrating factitious medical or psychiatric symptoms in order to get a tangible reward, such as narcotic drugs or disability payments, with the patients' awareness that they are lying and know what they want to achieve from their deceptions

Mall formula [mawl FOR-myoo-lah] method of calculating the age of a human embryo in days; calculated by taking the square root of the length from vertex to breech in centimeters, then multiplying by 100

malleolus [mal-EE-oh-lus] rounded distal projections of the distal tibia and fibula that comprise the ankle

malrotation [mal-roh-TAY-shun] rotation of a organ or structure in such a manner as to cut off function and/or blood supply

maltase [MAWL-tays] enzyme that converts maltose to glucose

mammary [MAM-ah-ree] pertaining to breast tissue or ducts

mandible [MAN-dih-bul] the bone of the lower jaw

-mania [MAY-nee-ah] *suffix*; indicating frenzy or a hyperexcited state

Mantoux test [man-TOO test] use of a four-pronged device to puncture the skin to deliver purified protein derivative from the mycobacterium tuberculosis to determine patient's exposure to tuberculosis

manubrium [mah-NYOO-bree-um] a triangular bone located at the most superior part of the sternum

marasmus [mah-RAZ-mus] chronic malnutrition caused by starvation, resulting in severe wasting of body tissues with: loss of subcutaneous fat; inelastic, wrinkled skin; loss of muscle tissue and strength; failure to grow; lethargy; and hypoproteinemia

masseter muscle [mas-SEE-ter MUS-sel] the muscle that closes the jaw and is used in chewing

mast- [mast] prefix; breast

mastication [mas-tih-KAY-shun] the process of chewing

mastoid [MASS-toyd] portion of the temporal bone of the skull located just behind and inferior to the ear

mastoidectomy [MASS-toy-DEK-toh-mee] surgical removal of the distal portion of the mastoid bone (mastoid process) and portions of the mastoid sinus; usually due to untreated otitis media

mastopexy [MAS-toh-peck-see] plastic surgery performed to correct drooping breasts to improve their look and form

maxilla [MAK-sil-ah] bone of the upper jaw

maxillofacial [MAK-sil-oh-FAY-shal] pertaining to the maxilla and upper face region

meatotomy [mee-ah-TOH-mee] enlargement of a passageway or channel by making an incision

meatus [ME-ayt-us] an opening or tunnel that connects internal and external surfaces

mechanical ventilation [meh-KAN-ih-kal ven-tih-LAY-shun] use of artificially supplied respirations using an automated respirator

Meckel's diverticulum [MEK-elz dy-ver-TIK-yoo-lum] a blind pouch that results when the omphalomesenteric duct, which connects the gut to the yolk sac during embryonic development, fails to atrophy

meconium [mee-KO-nee-um] first stool produced by newborn babies, which is characteristically greenish-black, thick, and sticky

medial [MEE-dee-al] going toward the middle

medial rectus muscle [MEE-dee-al REK-tus MUS-sel] muscle that moves the eye toward the midline

mediastinal nodes [med-ih-STIN-al nohdz] lymph tissue in the anterior chest

mediastinum [mee-dee-ah-STY-num] middle body cavity, midchest, directly above the diaphragm

medulla [meh-DOO-lah] innermost area of an organ or structure; for example, a lymph node or the kidney

medulla oblongata [meh-DOO-lah ob-long-GAH-tah] section of the brain stem that is continuous with the spinal cord

medullary cavity [MED-uhl-ar-ee KAV-ih-tee] the long cavity in the center of a long bone that contains yellow bone marrow

medullary rhythmicity area [MED-uhl-ar-ee rith-MIS-ih-tee AIR-ee-uh] brain region that regulates breathing patterns

medulloblastoma [meh-DOO-loh-blas-TOH-mah] a soft, infiltrating tumor of the external layer of cerebellum

mega- [meg-ah] prefix; large or oversized

megacolon [MEG-ah-koh-lon] condition of the colon with extreme dilation and hypertrophy

megakaryocyte [meg-ah-KAIR-ee-oh-site] a large cell normally found in the bone marrow that gives rise to platelets and has a multilobed nucleus

-megaly [meg-ah-lee] *suffix*; enlargement

meibomian glands [my-BOE-mee-an GLANZ] sebaceous glands at the edges of the eyelids that secrete sebum from their ducts

meiosis [my-OH-sis] division of a sex cell whereby the nucleus has 23 chromosomes

Meissner's plexus [MIS-nerz PLEK-sus] bundle of autonomic nerves located in the submucosa of the small intestine

melalgia [mel-AL-jee-ah] pain in the limbs from muscular sources

melagra [mel-AH-grah] pain in the limbs from neurological sources

melanemesis [mel-ahn-EM-eh-sis] vomitus with presence of blood in stomach contents due to bleeding ulcers

melanoma [mel-ah-NOH-mah] malignant tumor of melanocytes

melatonin [mel-ah-TOE-nin] hormone that is formed by the pineal gland and involved in circadian rhythms and bioregulation

melena [meh-LEE-nah] dark, tarry stools that contain digested blood due to bleeding from the esophagus or stomach

melenic [meh-LEH-nik] having the characteristic of dark, tarry stools

menarche [men-AR-kee] onset of regular menstrual cycle, with usual onset at approximately 13 years of age

Mendelsohn maneuver [MEN-del-son ma-NU-ver] a technique of swallowing that maintains voluntary muscular contraction for a few seconds at the highest position; used for management of swallowing disorders

Ménière's disease [men-YARZ dis-EEZ] a rare condition of the inner ear characterized by progressive hearing loss, sensation of pressure in the ear, tinnitus, and vertigo

meningioma [men-in-jee-OH-mah] a benign tumor of the coverings of the brain

meningocele [men-IN-goh-seel] protrusion of the meninges through bone, forming a filled cyst

meniscus [men-IS-kus] a crescent-shaped, fibrocartilaginous structure of the knee, acromioclavicular, and temporo-mandibular, and sternoclavicular joints

menopause [MEN-oh-pawz] termination of menses and ability to conceive

menorrhagia [men-oh-RAH-jee-ah] excessive uterine bleeding during menstruation

menorrhea [men-oh-REE-ah] normal menstruation

mental scotoma [MEN-tal sko-TOH-mah] inability to comprehend or demonstrate insight into a highly emotional subject, also known as an "emotional blind spot"

mentum [MEN-tum] chin

mesenteric [mez-en-TAIR-ik] pertaining to middle intestine attachment to the jejunum and iliac, the middle parts of the small intestine

-meso [mez-oh] *suffix*; middle

meta- [met-ah] *prefix*; change, going beyond normal development

metabolic syndrome [met-ah-BOL-ik SIN-drom] characteristics that increase the likelihood of development of heart disease, stroke, and diabetes whereby the individual possesses three out of five known risk factors (hypertension, abdominal obesity, elevated triglycerides, low HDL, and elevated fasting glucose)

metabolism [meh-TAB-oh-lih-zim] entire transformation of energy and chemicals occurring within living cells, consisting of anabolism and catabolism

metacarpal [MET-ah-KAR-pal] the five bones that make up the hand

metaphysis [met-ah-FIH-sis] portion of a bone where growth occurs, situated between the diaphysis and epiphysis

metastasize [met-TAS-tah-size] spreading of malignant cells to surrounding tissues and other parts of the body though the blood and lymph

metatarsal bones [met-ah-TAR-sal bohnz] the five long bones of the foot

-meter [mee-ter] *suffix*; instrument used for measurement

metered dose inhaler [MEE-terd dose in-HAIL-er] medical device used to deliver a specific quantity of aerosolized medication to the airway

methicillin-resistant *Staphylococcus aureus* [meth-ah-SIL-in-ree-SIS-tant staf-il-oh-KOK-kus ar-REE-us] clustered bacteria that are not affected by the antibiotic class of methicillin

metopic [mee-TOH-pik] relating to the anterior portion of the cranium or forehead

metratonia [mee-trah-TOH-nee-ah] atony of the uterine wall following childbirth

metritis [mee-TRY-tis] inflammation of the uterus

metrorrhagia [mee-troh-RAY-jee-ah] uterine bleeding at times other than the regular menstrual period

-metry [meh-tree] *suffix*; process of measurement

micrencephaly [my-kren-SEF-ah-lee] abnormally small size of the brain

micro- [my-crow] *prefix*; small

microcytic anemia [MY-kroh-SYT-ik ah-NEE-mee-ah] anemia where the average size of circulating erythrocytes is smaller than normal

microgram [MY-kro-gram] unit of measurement equaling one-millionth of a gram

microhepatia [my-kro-hee-PAT-ee-ah] abnormally small-sized liver

micronodular goiter [MY-kro-NOHD-yoo-lar GOY-tur] enlargement of the thyroid gland with small nodules that give the tissue a slightly more granular appearance than normal tissue

microphobia [my-kro-FOH-bee-ah] fear of germs

micturition [mik-too-RIH-shun] urination

micturition syncope [mik-too-RIH-shun SIN-koh-pee] sudden loss of consciousness during urination; most often observed in men

midbrain [mid-BRAYN] the middle region of the brain stem responsible for auditory and visual reflex centers

midsagittal [mid-SAJ-ih-tal] direction of going from front to back of body

migraine headache [MY-grane HED-ayk] periodic and severe pain in the head associated with vertigo, photosensitivity, scintillation, nausea, and vomiting

Minamata disease [min-ah-MAW-tah dis-EEZ] neurological disorder due to methyl mercury intoxication resulting from eating fish contaminated with mercury waste in the water; symptoms include peripheral sensory loss, dysarthria, tremors, ataxia, and hearing and vision loss

miosis [mi-OH-sis] abnormal constriction of the iris muscle to decrease the size of the pupil and limit the amount of light entering the eye; associated with stroke, head trauma, and eyedrops containing agents that deactivate acetylcholinesterase

mitochondrion [my-toh-KON-dree-on] a rod- or oval-shaped cytoplasmic organelle that produces energy within the cell by the production of adenosine triphosphate (ATP)

mitosis [my-TOH-sis] the division of cells in the body in which the 46 chromosomes in the nucleus duplicate and then split, creating two identical cells, each with 46 chromosomes

mitral insufficiency [MIGH-tral in-suh-FISH-en-see] faulty sealing of the bicuspid valve, causing backflow of blood into the atrium from the ventricle

mitral stenosis [MIGH-tral steh-NOH-sis] narrowing of the mitral valve opening, causing impaired blood flow

mitral valve [MIGH-tral valv] the valve closing the blood flow between the left atrium and left ventricle of the heart; also called the bicuspid valve due to having two cusps (anterior and posterior)

mitral valve prolapse [MIGH-tral valv PRO-laps] faulty sealing of the bicuspid valve due to chordae tendineae failure that permits backward flow of blood

mixed hearing loss [myxt HEER-ing loss] reduced hearing acuity due to a combination of sensorineural and conductive pathology

Mohs surgery [MOHZ SUR-jer-ee] microscopically controlled cancer surgery

molluscum contagiosum [mo-LUS-kum con-tay-gee-OH-sum] a sexually transmitted disease of the skin caused by infection with a virus from the *Poxviridae* family; typical presentation is the appearance of small, pearl-shaped epidermal growths on or around the genitals

mono- [mon-oh] *prefix*; single

mononucleosis [mon-oh-nyoo-klee-OH-sis] condition of having abnormally high numbers of mononuclear leukocytes in the blood, due to infection by the Epstein-Barr virus

monophasia [mon-oh-FAY-zee-ah] speech disorder characterized by the inability to state anything but one word or phrase in a repetitious fashion

monoplegia [mon-oh-PLEE-jee-uh] paralysis of a single limb

monorchism [mon-OR-kizm] condition of having only one descended testicle

monozygotic [mon-oh-zy-GOT-ik] twins or multiple births originating from a single zygote that separates early in development; resulting individuals have identical genetic makeup

mora reflex [MOR-ah REE-fleks] Involuntary response in infants, present from birth to six months; when startled by noise or change in position, the arms extend and then move toward the chest

morbidity [mohr-BID-it-ee] sickness, or state of disease

-morph [morf] *suffix*; form or shape

morphology [mor-FAWL-oh-jee] classification of organisms by structure and form

motile [MOE-til] pertaining to movement

-motor [MOE-tor] *suffix*; something that produces movement

mucocutaneous lymph node syndrome [myoo-koh-kyoo-TAN-ee-us lymf nohd SIN-drom] a febrile illness in children marked by fever, rashes, lymphadenopathy, and cardiac complications; also known as Kawasaki disease

mucolytic [myoo-koh-LIH-tik] drug(s) used to break up thick mucus so it can be coughed up

mucopurulent [myoo-koh-PUR-uu-lent] mucus with pus, usually indicative of chronic obstructive pulmonary disease (COPD)

mucosa [myoo-KOH-sah] mucous membrane

multi- [mul-tie] *prefix*; many

multi-infarct dementia [MUL-tie-IN-farkt dee-MEN-shee-ah] decreased cognitive functioning due to many small vascular occlusions in the brain

multipara [mul-tih-PAR-ah] a woman who has carried more than one fetus to the point of viability

multiple sclerosis (MS) [MUL-tih-pul skle-ROH-sis] disease of the central nervous system characterized by the demyelination and deterioration of the myelin sheath of nerve fibers with episodes of neurological dysfunction (exacerbation) followed by recovery (remission)

Münchhausen by proxy [mun-CHOW-zen by PRAWX-see] patient creates illness in another person, often a child or other dependent individual, by inducing physical symptoms with drugs or by contaminating laboratory tests, in order to gain attention as the sacrificing, loving caregiver

Münchhausen syndrome [mun-CHOW-zen SIN-drom] patients with this disorder demonstrate factitious medical or psychiatric symptoms with awareness that they are lying, but are unaware of the underlying need for attention, resulting in numerous tests, treatments, and surgeries

murmur [MER-mer] abnormal blowing or roaring heart sounds heard on auscultation, caused by defective valves or chambers of the heart

muscle biopsy [MUS-sel BY-op-see] tissue sample taken for skeletal muscle for evaluation to assist in diagnosis of myopathy

muscular dystrophies [MUS-ku-lar DIS-troh-feez] hereditary diseases marked by muscle-cell degeneration

muscular insertion [MUS-ku-lar in-SER-shun] point of attachment to bone at the site of greatest movement; opposite of muscular origin

muscular origin [MUS-ku-lar OR-ih-jin] point of attachment to a stationary or nearly stationary bone of the skeleton; opposite of muscular insertion

musculature [MUS-kyoo-lah-tchur] the muscles of the body or the muscles in a particular part of the body

myalgia [migh-AL-jee-uh] muscle pain

myasthenia gravis [migh-as-THEEN-ee-uh GRAV-is] an immunologic neuromuscular disorder characterized by fluctuating muscular strength, poor activity tolerance, and notable weakness of the oculofacial and proximal limb muscle groups

mycosis fungoides [my-KOH-sis fung-GOYD-eez] cutaneous T-cell lymphoma characterized by irregular shaped nodules and plaques on the trunk that spread to lymph nodes and internal organs

mydriasis [mih-DRY-eh-sis] dilation of the pupil

myelin [MIGH-e-lin] white, fatty substance that forms the nerve sheath

myelin sheath [MIGH-e-lin sheeth] a fatty substance surrounding some neurons that acts as an electrical insulator, increasing the speed of nerve impulse transmission

myelitis [migh-eh-LYE-tis] inflammation of the spinal cord

myelocyte [MIGH-eh-loh-site] an immature cell in the bone marrow that produces leukocytes

myelogenous leukemia [MIGH-eh-LAWJ-eh-nus loo-KEE-mee-ah] hematological disorder characterized by proliferation of myelopoietic cells and grossly increased numbers of immature and mature granulocytes in the blood and organs

myelogram [MIGH-eh-loh-gram] radiographic imagery of the spine and spinal nerves

myelosuppression [migh-eh-loh-su-PRESH-un] decreased production of blood cells by the bone marrow

myocardial contusion [migh-oh-KAR-dee-ul kon-TOO-shun] injury resulting from a strong, blunt force against the chest wall that injures the heart muscle, disrupting blood flow to areas of the heart muscle

myocardial infarction [migh-oh-KAR-dee-ul in-FARK-shun] necrosis of a portion of cardiac muscle caused by partial or complete occlusion of one or more coronary arteries; also known as heart attack

myocardiorrhaphy [migh-oh-KAR-dee-or-RAF-ee] surgical repair of the muscle of the heart by suturing

myocarditis [migh-oh-kar-DYE-tis] inflammation of the myocardium due to microbial infection, toxin exposure, or chronic cocaine use

myoclonus [MIGH-oh-KLOH-nus] rapid, intense contractions of a muscle group that is usually indicative of a central nervous system lesion

myofascial pain syndrome [migh-oh-FAY-shul payn SIN-drom] chronic discomfort in muscles and soft tissues surrounding joints; also known as fibromyalgia syndrome

myofibrils [migh-oh-FIGH-brilz] filaments in muscle cytoplasm

myoglobin [migh-oh-GLOH-bin] a ferrous globin complex consisting of one heme molecule containing one iron molecule attached to a single globin chain

myopathy [migh-OP-uth-ee] any disease of the muscles

myopia [migh-OH-pee-ah] refractive error of the eye resulting in inability to focus on objects at a distance; also known as nearsightedness

myositis [migh-oh-SIGH-tis] muscle inflammation

myotonia [migh-oh-TOH-nee-ah] a type of dystonia characterized by an inability to relax a muscle

myringa [migh-RIN-guh] tympanic membrane; also known as the eardrum

myringotomy [mir-ing-GOT-oh-me] surgical process of cutting into the eardrum to remove fluid from the middle ear

myxedema [miks-eh-DEE-mah] form of hypothyroidism which occurs in adults with decreased T4 and thyrotropin hormone production; key symptom is water retention; treatment is usually by administration of synthetic T4 levothyroxine sodium or Synthroid

narcolepsy [NAR-koh-lep-see] a sleep disorder characterized by the frequent, sudden, uncontrollable need to sleep and by temporary muscular paralysis

nares [NAIR-eez] the external cartilage of the nose

nasal [NAY-zal] pertaining to the nose

nasal ala [NAY-zal AYE-lah] flared cartilage on each side of the nostril

nasogastric tube [nay-zoh-GAS-rik TOOBE] a small-caliber tube inserted in the nose and leading to the stomach for feeding or suctioning

nasolacrimal duct [NAY-soh-LAK-rih-mal DUHKT] a tube that carries tears from the lacrimal sac to the inside of the nose

-nate [nate] *suffix;* born

nausea [NAW-zee-uh] an unsettled feeling in the stomach with the urge to vomit

navicular [nah-VIK-yoo-lar] bones of the wrist and ankle that are shaped like a boat

nebulizer [NEB-yoo-lye-zur] a device used for producing fine mist for inhalation for the purpose of delivery of medications directly into the lung

necatoriasis [nee-ka-toe-RY-ah-sis] infestation with a parasitic hookworm

necropsy [NEK-rop-see] examination of a body to determine the cause of death; autopsy

necrosis [ne-KRO-sis] death of living cells or tissue; gangrene

necrotizing fasciitis [NEK-roh-ty-zing fas-ee-FYE tis] an infection that spreads extremely rapidly and travels through tissue along superficial and deep planes; treatment includes aggressive surgical debridement and antibiotics in order to prevent death

needle biopsy [NEE-del BY-op-see] procedure of obtaining a deep-tissue sample for examination by piercing a lesion with a needle and withdrawing the tissue in the lumen of the needle

negative pressure ventilation [NEG-ah-tiv PRESH-sur ven-tih-LAY-shun] mechanical support of respiration using chambers that encase the body to create intermittent subatmospheric pressure to extend the chest outward and fill the lungs

neo- [nee-oh] *prefix*; new

neologism [nee-AWL-oh-jizm] fabricated words with meaning known only to the speaker; sometimes associated with schizophrenia or Tourette's disorder

neoplasm [NEE-oh-plaz-im] new growth of cells that may be malignant or benign

neoplastic [NEE-oh-plas-tik] pertaining to a growth of tissue which may be benign or malignant

neoplastic heart syndrome [NEE-oh-plas-tik hart SIN-drom] absence or stenosis of the mitral and aortic valves associated with an abnormally small left ventricle and aortic arch, possibly due to genetic factors

nephrectomy [nef-REK-toh-mee] surgical removal of a kidney

nephritis [nef-RYE-tis] inflammation of the nephrons or kidney inflammation as seen in acute nephritis, glomerulonephritis, and interstitial nephritis

nephroblastoma [NEF-roh-blas-TOH-mah] a rapidly developing, malignant tumor of the kidney occurring in children with deletion of chromosomes 11 and 16; also called Wilms tumor

nephrolithotomy [NEF-roh-lith-AWT-oh-mee] surgical procedure in which a small incision is made in the skin for the use of a fiberoptic scope to remove renal calculi

nephropathy [neh-FROP-ah-thee] kidney disease

nephropexy [NEF-roh-pek-see] surgical fixation to secure a floating or ptotic kidney

nephroptosis [nef-rop-TOE-sis] moveable or downward displacement of the kidney

nephrosis [nef-ROH-sis] degenerative renal condition characterized by damage to the renal tubules without inflammation; also called nephrotic syndrome

nephrotic syndrome [nef-ROT-ik SIN-drom] degenerative renal lesions resulting from damage to the basement membrane of the glomeruli; commonly seen as a complication from systemic diseases such as diabetes mellitus, systemic lupus erythematosus, and multiple myeloma

nephrotoxic [nef-roh-TOK-sik] poisonous or destructive to the kidney

nerve block [NERV blok] injection of anesthetic into peripheral nerves or nerve trunks to interrupt sensation

nerve cell fiber [nerv sel FY ber] linked neurons that transmit electrical and chemical messages between the body and central nervous system

nerve decompression [nerv dee-kom-PRESH-un] surgical intervention to relieve pressure on a nerve by excision of constricting bands of tissue or by enlarging the bony canal

nerve impulse [NERV IM-puls] transmission of stimuli to or from the central nervous system

nerve tract [NERV trakt] a group of nerve fibers that are either afferent or efferent in their function

nervus frontalis [NERV-us fron-TAH-lis] branch of the occipitalis nerve that divides in the orbit into the supraorbital and supratrochlear nerves

neural tunics [NEW-rul TEW-niks] the layer of the eye containing the retina

neuralgia [nu-RAL-jee-ah] severe pain along the course of a nerve

neurectomy [nyoo-REK-toh-mee] partial or complete surgical excision or resection of a nerve

neurilemma [NU-ri-LEM-ah] membrane forming the myelin sheath

neuroblastoma [NYOO-roh-blas-TOH-ma] malignant neoplasm with proliferation of immature nerve cells, most often diagnosed in infants and children

neurofibrillary tangles [nyoor-oh-FIH-brih-lar-ee TAN-gelz] misshaped filaments on the surface of the brain associated with Alzheimer's-type dementia

neurofibromatosis [NU-roh-fi-broh-mah-TOH-sis] a group of genetic diseases that affect cell growth of neural tissues, with multiple subcutaneous tumors and tumors of the eighth cranial nerve

neuroganglion [nyoo-roh-GAN-glee-on] cysts containing fluid within a fibrous capsule attached to a tendon sheath of the hands, wrists, or feet

neurogenic bladder [new-roh-JEN-ik BLAD-der] urinary bladder dysfunction including incomplete emptying, urinary retention, and frequent infection resulting from impaired nervous system functioning

neuroglia [nyoo-ROG-lee-uh] supportive, non-nerve tissues of the peripheral and central nervous system

neurohypophysis [nyoo-roh-high-POF-ih-SIS] a neurological structure at the base of the hypothalamus including the infundibulum and the posterior lobe of the pituitary gland

neuroleptic [nyoo-roh-LEP-tik] category of pharmacological agents that treat psychotic symptoms by reducing the amount of dopamine in the brain

neuroleptic malignant syndrome [nyoo-roh-LEP-tik mah-LIG-nant SIN-drom] a potentially fatal complication following administration of antipsychotic medications; characterized by severe hyperthermia, confusion, gross diaphoresis, renal failure, and seizures

neurology [nyoo-RAWL-oh-jee] branch of medicine that deals with disorders of the central and peripheral nervous systems

neurolysis [nyoo-ROL-eye-is] cutting or freeing nerve tissue from inflammatory adhesions

neuromuscular junction [NYOO-roh-MUS-ku-lar JUNKT-shun] location of connection of nerves to muscle tissues

neuron [NYOO-ron] the functional unit of the nervous system responsible for conducting impulses; includes the axion, cell body, and dendrites

neurosis [nyoo-ROH-sis] psychiatric disorder that affects coping which results in maladaptive behaviors but does not prevent functioning

neurosyphilis [nyoo-roh-SIF-ih-lis] infection of the central nervous system with *Treponema pallidum*, causing dementia and other degenerative changes; may be asymptomatic or involve the meninges and vascular structures in the brain and/or spinal cord

neurotransmitter [nyoo-roh-TRANS-mit-er] any one of numerous chemicals that modify or result in the transmission of nerve impulses between synapses

neutropenia [NYOO-troh-PEE-nee-uh] condition of diminished quantity of white blood cells in the circulating blood

neutrophil [NYOO-troh-fil] a mature white blood cell formed in the bone marrow

nitroglycerin [nigh-troh-GLIS-er-in] a fast-acting vasodilator drug

noci- [noh-sih] *prefix*; injury; experiencing or producing pain

nociceptor [noh-sih-SEP-tor] a peripheral nerve responsible for perception of pain

nodule [NOD-uhl] a small lymph node; small circumscribed swelling

non- [non] *prefix*; not

noncontributory [non-kon-TRIB-yew-tor-ee] not involved in bringing on the condition or disease

nondisplaced fracture [non-dis-PLAYSD FRAK-shur] a broken bone that remains in the normal anatomical alignment

nontoxic goiter [non-TAWK-sik GOY-ter] thyroid enlargement without excessive production of thyroid hormone

nonunion [non-yoon-yun] a fractured bone that fails to heal properly

noradrenaline [nor-ah-DREN-ah-lin] adrenal medulla hormone; norepinephrine

norepinephrine [nor-ep-ih-NEF-rin] adrenal medulla hormone; noradrenaline

normal flora [NOR-mal FLOOR-ah] bacteria that are expected and healthy in the body

normal sinus rhythm [NOR-mal SY-nus RITH-em] heart rate and electrical conduction originating from the sinoatrial node

normochromasia [nor-moh-KRO-may-see-uh] attribute of tissues or cells that have average staining ability

normochromic [NOR-moh-krom-ik] pertaining to red blood cells in which the amount of hemoglobin is normal and therefore have a normal red color

Norwood procedure [NOR-wood pro-SEE-jur] surgical creation of a conduit between the aorta and pulmonary artery to increase blood flow to the aorta

nosocomial [nos-oh-KOH-mee-al] disease caused by exposure to a pathogen in the hospital setting

nuclear scan [nu-klee-ar skan] diagnostic technique making use of radiopharmaceutical injection, inhalation, or ingestion for the purpose of studying the structure and function of an area of the body or organ

nuclease [NYOO-klee-ays] an enzyme that breaks down nucleic acid

nucleic acid [NYOO-klee-ic AS-id] chemicals that carry genetic information in the form of deoxyribonucleic acid (DNA) and ribonucleic acid (RNA)

nucleus pulposus [NEW-klee-us pul-POH-sus] center of the intervertebral disc

nulligravida [nul-ih-GRAV-ih-dah] a woman who has never been pregnant

nutrient foramen [NEW-tree-ent fo-RAY-men] opening in bone through which nerves or blood vessels pass

nystagmus [nys-TAG-mus] involuntary rhythmic ocular movements, particularly when looking to the side; each back-and-forth motion is known as a beat

O

obesity [oh-BEE-sit-tee] weight 20 percent above the recommended weight for sex and height

obfuscation [OB-fyoo-SKAY-shun] mental confusion associated with gross sedation and brain disorders

obicularis oris muscle [oh-BIK-yoo-lar-is OR-is MUS-sel] facial muscle that circles the mouth

oblique fissure [oh-BLEEK FISH-sur] anatomical landmark of the right lung

oblique fracture [oh-BLEEK FRAK-shur] a slanting-angle break in bone

obliteration [ob-LIT-er-AY-shun] loss of body function or part due to surgical intervention, disease, or degenerative condition

obsession [awb-SESH-un] constant, persistent, uncontrollable thoughts associated with anxiety and psychotic disorders

obsessive-compulsive disorder [awb-SESS-iv-kom-PUL-sive dis-OR-der] psychiatric illness characterized by persistent, uncontrollable thoughts that cause anxiety and compel the patient to perform excessive, repetitive activities causing incapacity

obstetrics [ob-STEH-triks] branch of medicine focused on the care of women during pregnancy, delivery, and the postpartum period

obstipated [ob-stih-PAY-ted] severe, unrelieved constipation

obstructive cholangitis [ob-STRUK-tiv koh-lan-JY-tis] an acute or chronic inflammation of the bile ducts due to cirrhosis or gallstones

obstructive jaundice [ob-STRUK-tiv JON-dis] yellowish discoloration of skin and sclera due to a gallstone or other pathology blocking the flow of bile in the bile ducts (obstructive cholangitis)

obstructive shock [ob-STRUK-tiv shok] condition that occurs when a blockage of the main bloodstream interferes with tissue perfusion; possible causes include compression vena cava, pericardial tamponade, and pulmonary embolism

obtund [ob-TUND] to dull or decrease perception of pain

obturating embolism [OB-too-RAY-ting EM-boh-lizm] complete occlusion of a blood vessel by a clot or plaque

obturator foramen [AWB-too-RAY-tor fo-RAY-men] a large opening in the ischium that is covered by a fibrous membrane and is a point of attachment for some muscles of the hip

occipital bone [ok-SIP-ih-tal bone] osseous formation of the posterior base of the cranium

occipital lobe [ok-SIP-ih-tal lohb] most distal section of the brain; involved in vision

occipitalis muscle [ok-SIP-it-tal-is MUS-sel] muscle that retracts and tenses scalp

occlusion [oh-KLOO-zhun] the action of closing off or being closed; relationship between upper and lower teeth of the jaw

occult [oh-KULT] hidden, not observable by the naked eye; often used in reference to bleeding in the gastrointestinal tract

occult blood [oh-KULT blud] hidden blood in stool that is not visible to the unaided eye

occupational disease [OK-yoo-PAY-shun-al diz-EEZ] health alteration due to exposure or activities associated with work activity or job

octa- [ok-tah] *prefix*; eight

oculogyric crisis [ok-yoo-loh-JYE-rik KRY-sis] acute spasm and involuntary deviation or fixation of the eyes in an upward gaze; associated with dystonia from antipsychotic or antiemetic medications

oculomotor nerve [OK-yoo-loh-MOH-tor nerv] the third cranial nerve, which functions primarily to send impulses to the muscles of the eyes and eyelids in order to direct movement

oculus dexter (OD) [OK-yoo-lus DEKS-ter] right eye

oculus sinister (OS) [OK-yoo-lus SIN-is-ter] left eye

odontoid process [oh-DON-toyd PRAW-sess] a toothlike formation on the second vertebra upon which the head rotates

odynophagia [oh-DIN-oh-FAY-jee-ah] difficult or painful eating or swallowing

-oid [oyd] *suffix*; similar to

-ole [ohl] *suffix*; small

olecranon process [oh-LEK-rah-non PRAW-sess] the curved segment of the ulna commonly referred to as the elbow

olfaction [ol-FAK-shun] sense of smell or act of smelling

olfactory aura [ol-FAK-toh-ree AW-rah] subjective sensation of smell experienced just prior to the onset of seizure activity

olig- [oh-lig] *prefix*; inadequate number; few; too little

oligodipsia [oh-lig-oh-DIP-see-uh] diminished thirst sensation

oligopnea [oh-li-GOP-nee-ah] infrequent breathing that causes less oxygen to enter the lungs

oligospermia [oh-lig-oh-SPER-mee-uh] decreased quantity of sperm in the ejaculate

oliguria [oh-LIG-ur-ree-ah] scant or inadequate urine production

-ologist [ol-oh-gist] *suffix*; one who practices a specialty

-oma [oh-mah] *suffix*; tumor

omo- [oh-mo] *prefix*; shoulder or upper arm

omphal- [om-fal] prefix; pertaining to navel

omphaloceles [oom-fal-OH-seelz] congenital malformations in which intra-abdominal contents protrude through the umbilical cord

onch- [onk] *prefix*; fingernails

oncology [on-KOL-oh-jee] a branch of medicine focused on the treatment of cancers

onocryptosis [on-oh-krip-TOH-sis] ingrown fingernail or toenail

onychia [oh-NIK-ee-ah] inflammation of the nail matrix or bed

onycholysis [on-ih-KOL-ih-sis] loosening of the nail from the nail bed

onychomycosis [on-ih-koh-migh-KOH-sis] fungal infection of the nail

onychophagia [on-ih-KOF-ah-jee-ah] nail-biting

oo- [yoo] *prefix*; ovum or egg

oophorectomy [oh-oof-oh-REK-toh-mee] surgical removal of one or both ovaries

oophorocystectomy [oh-OOF-oh-roh-sis-TEK-tom-ee] surgical removal of an ovarian cyst

oophorragia [oh-off-oh-RAY-jee-ah] hemorrhaging from the ovary

open reduction and internal fixation (ORIF) [OH-pen ree-DUK-shun and in-TER-nal fik-SAY-shun] surgical treatment to stabilize a complex fracture where an incision is made at the fracture site and the fracture is realigned using screws, nails, or plates to hold the fracture fragments in correct anatomical alignment

ophthalmoscope [op-THAL-moh-skop] an instrument used to examine the retina and interior structures of the eye

-opia [oh-pee-ah] *suffix*; condition of vision

opiate [OH-pee-ayt] narcotic drugs used for the treatment of pain

opisth- [op-isth] *prefix*; backward

opponens pollicis muscle [op-POH-nenz POL-ih-sis MUS-sel] muscle of the hand that pulls the thumb across the palm to enable a pinch-type grasp

opportunistic infection [awp-or-too-NIS-tik in-FEK-shun] disease caused by bacteria or viruses due to immunosuppression

oppositional defiant disorder [AWP-ih-SIH-shun-al dee-FY-ant dis-OR-der] persistent, aggressive behavior (fighting, arguing, provoking, annoying), defiance of and refusal to obey rules, disrespect for authority figures, with anger, stubbornness, and touchiness

-opsy [op-see] *suffix*; to view

optic [AWP-tik] pertaining to vision or the orbit

optic chiasm [AWP-tik KY-ah-zim] area in the brain where parts of the right and left optic nerves cross and join the other optic nerve

optic disc [AWP-tik disk] a small circular portion of the retina where the optic nerve passes through and does not have visual capacity

optic nerve [AWP-tik nerv] cranial nerve II, which carries nerve impulses of visual images from the rods and cones of the retina to the visual cortex in the brain

optician [op-TISH-an] expert who fills prescriptions for eyeglasses and contact lenses

optometrist [op-TOM-eh-trist] specialist in the testing of visual function and in the diagnosis and nonsurgical treatment of eye conditions

oral antidiabetic [OR-al AN-tee-dye-uh-BET-ik] pharmacological agents used to decrease blood glucose levels

oral cavity [OR-al KAV-ih-tee] the mouth, inclusive of the teeth, mucosa, and lips

oral cholecystography [OR-al KOH-lee-sis-TOH-grah-fee] radiological procedure that uses orally ingested tablets of radiopaque contrast dye

orbicularis muscle [oh-bik-yoo-LAIR-is MUS-sel] muscle that closes the eyelid

orbicularis oculi muscle [or-bik-yoo-LAIR-is OK-yoo-lye MUS-sel] muscle that circles the eye

orbicularis oris muscle [or-bik-yoo-LAIR-is OR-is MUS-sel] muscle that compresses the lips

orbit [OR-bit] round circuit, pertaining to the eye or bony socket in the cranium that surrounds all but the anterior portion of the eye

orchidoplasty [OR-kid-oh-PLAS-tee] surgical reconstruction of a testicle

organ of Corti [OR-gan of KOR-tee] the long, spiral-shaped structure that extends along the floor of the cochlear duct and is stimulated by sound waves

oropharynx [OR-oh-FAIR-inks] region of the throat located between the soft palate and the epiglottis

-orrhea [or-ree-ah] *suffix;* excessive discharge or flow

-orrheixis [or-reeks-is] *suffix;* rupture

orthopedist [OR-tho-PEE-dist] physician who diagnoses and treats patients with skeletal and muscular disorders

orthopnea [or-THOP-nee-uh] lung disease that causes the patient to assume an upright or semi-upright position in order to breathe and sleep comfortably; dyspnea and congestion in the lungs occur when lying down

orthosis [or-THOH-sis] orthopedic device such as a brace, splint, or collar used to immobilize or correct an orthopedic problem; often custom-made to fit the patient's specific measurements

orthotonos [or-THOT-oh-nus] type of tetanic spasm where the limbs, neck, and trunk are held in a rigid, straight line

os [OS] bone

os calis [os KAL-is] bone of the heel

os pubis [os PYOO-bis] pubic bone; one of three bones that fuse together to form the hip bone

oscheo- [os-kee-oh] *prefix*; pertaining to the scrotum

-ose [ohs] *suffix*; carbohydrate

-osis [oh-sis] *suffix*; condition or increased

osmo- [oz-moh] *prefix*; pertaining to odor, smell

osmolarity [oz-moh-LAIR-ih-tee] total concentration of dissolved substances in a solution; osmotic concentration

osmotic pressure [oz-MOT-ik PRESH-sur] part of the blood pressure that is due to plasma proteins; also known as blood colloid osmotic pressure

osphresio- [os-free-see-oh] *prefix*; pertaining to odor or sense of smell

osseous [AW-see-us] pertaining to bone

ossicles [AWS-ih-kulz] three tiny bones in each ear: malleus, incus, and stapes; also called the ossicular chain due to their arrangement in a row

ossification [AWS-ih-fih-KAY-shun] a process occurring during childhood until cartilaginous tissue is gradually replaced by bony tissue

osteo- [ost-ee-oh] *prefix*; pertaining to bone

osteoarthritis [AWS-tee-oh-ar-THRY-tis] degenerative joint disease characterized by deterioration of articular cartilage and bone hypertrophy

osteoblast [AWS-tee-oh-blast] mesodermal cells capable of producing new bone tissue

O

osteochondrosis [os-tee-kon-DROH-sis] degeneration and necrosis of the growth center of bones

osteoclasis [os-tee-oh-KLAY-sis] surgical fracture or rebreaking of a bone

osteoclasts [AWS-tee-oh-klasts] cells that break down areas of old or damaged bone

osteodysplasty [AWS-tee-oh-DIS-plas-tee] generalized skeletal dysplasia with prominent forehead and small mandible; irregular ribbon-like constrictions of the ribs and tubular bones demonstrated on x-rays

osteogenesis imperfecta [os-tee-oh-JEN-ee-sis im-pur-FEK-tah] brittle-bone disease characterized by sustaining multiple fractures throughout life from minimal trauma

osteoma [os-tee-OH-mah] a benign tumor of the bone

osteomalacia [os-tee-oh-mah-LAY-shee-ah] softening of the bone due to vitamin D deficiency in adults

osteomyelitis [AWS-tee-oh-my-LIE-tis] inflammation of the bone and bone marrow

osteophyte [AWS-tee-oh-fite] formation of bone fragments in the joint due to inflammation

osteoporosis [AWS-tee-oh poh-ROH-sis] loss of bone structure when the rate of resorption exceeds new bone formation; results in demineralized bone that is at risk for fractures

osteosarcoma [OS-tee-oh-sar-KOH-mah] malignant bone tumor that occurs predominantly in adolescents and is usually located at the metaphysis of the distal femur, proximal tibia, or proximal humerus

osteotome [AWS-tee-oh-tohm] a surgical tool used to cut bone

osteotomy [os-tee-OT-oh-mee] surgical incision into bone

otalgia [oh-TAL-jee-ah] earache

otitis media [oh-TYE-tis ME-dee-ah] inflammation of the middle ear

Glossary

oto- [oh-toh] *prefix*; pertaining to ear or auditory function

otolaryngologist [oh-toh-lar-in-GAWL-oh-jist] physician who practices the specialty of ear, nose, and throat disorders; also known as ENT specialists

-otomy [ot-oh-mee] *suffix*; to cut or incise

otoplasty [OH-toh-plas-tee] surgical correction of deformities of the external ear

otorhinolaryngology [oh-toh-ry-noh-lar-in-GOL-oh-jee] branch of medicine focused on the function and treatment of ear, nose, and larynx disorders

otorrhea [oh-toh-REE-ah] discharge from the ear

otosclerosis [oh-toh-skle-ROH-sis] decreased function or mobility of bones of the inner ear and the oval window, causing conductive loss

otoscope [OH-toh-skop] an instrument that provides light and magnification for viewing the external auditory canal

-ous [us] *suffix*; possessing or full of; pertaining to

oval window [OH-val WIN-doh] opening in the temporal bone between the middle ear and the vestibule of the inner ear which is covered by the end of the stapes

ovarian cyst [oh-VAR-ree-an SIST] abnormal cystic growth on the ovary comprised of a closed sac containing fluid, semifluid, or solid material

oviduct [OH-vih-dukt] the fallopian tube

oximeter [ok-SIM-ee-ter] instrument used to measure the concentration of hemoglobin in the blood

oxy- [ok-see] *prefix*; referring to oxygen; alternate meaning: sharp, keen, acute, or pungent

oxygenated [OK-see-Jen-ay-ted] having attached oxygen

oxyhemoglobin [OK-see-hee-moe-GLO-bin] oxygen molecules combine with the hemoglobin in red blood cells in the blood to form the compound oxyhemoglobin, transporting oxygen in the blood

oxytocia [OK-see-toh-see-ah] rapid labor

oxytocin [OK-see-TOH-sin] an agent that is administered to stimulate uterine contractions and accelerate delivery of a fetus

oxytocin challenge test [OK-see-TOH-sin CHAL-enj test] infusion of intravenous oxytocin to stimulate contractions

P

P wave [PEE wayv] section of the electrocardiogram (ECG) showing atrial depolarization

pacemaker [PAYS-may-ker] natural or artificial regulatory mechanism of rate of an activity; often used in relation to heart contraction

pachy- [pak-ee] *prefix*; profuse

pachymeningitis [PAK-ee-men-in-JY-tis] inflammation of the dura mater of the brain

pacing catheter [PAY-sing KATH-eh-ter] a cardiac catheter with electrodes at the end that is inserted into the patient's right ventricle to artificially regulate heart rhythm

Paget's disease [PAJ-ets dis-EEZ] a disorder characterized by increased bone resorption and formation, causing thickening and softening of bones

palinopsia [pal-ih-NOP-see-uh] abnormal experience of recurrent visual hallucinations

palliative care [PAL-ee-ah-tiv kair] use of therapies intended to comfort and support those with short life expectancies, focused primarily on symptom management rather than curative goals

pallidotomy [pal-ih-DOT-oh-mee] surgical destruction of the globus pallidus in the brain to decrease involuntary movements associated with Parkinson's disease

pallor [PAL-or] unnatural lightness in color of skin due to lack of blood supply to tissue

palmar grasp reflex [PAL-mar grasp REE-fleks] a primitive reflex present from birth to three months of age, triggered by placing a finger across the infant's palm and eliciting a strong grip around the finger

palpation [pal-PAY-shun] using the fingers to touch or press on the body surface to detect masses, enlargement, edema, or tenderness

palpebra [PAL-peh-bra] eyelid; may be further defined as superior or inferior to denote the upper or lower lid

palpitation [pal-plh-TAY-shun] sensation of irregular, strong, or fluttering heartbeat in the chest or neck

pan- [pan] *prefix*; all

pancolectomy [pan-koh-LEK-toh-mee] surgical removal of the entire colon

pancreas [PAN-kree-as] organ with endocrine and exocrine functions

pancreatectomy [pan-kree-ah-TEK-toh-mee] surgical excision of part or all of the pancreas

pancreatic islets [PAN-kree-at-ik EYE-lets] endocrine cells of the pancreas

pancreatitis [pan-kree-ah-TYE-tis] inflammation of the pancreas

pancreatography [pan-kree-ah-TOG-rah-fee] visualization of the pancreas using endoscopy and x-rays after injection of a radiopaque contrast medium into the duct of Wirsung

pancytopenia [pan-sy-toh-PEE-nee-uh] gross deficiency in all components of the blood

panic disorder [PAN-ik dis-OR-der] sudden episodes of severe, overwhelming anxiety without an identifiable cause; patients often report feeling that they are choking or dying of a heart attack

pant- [pant] *prefix*; all or the whole of something

Papanicolaou test [pa-pa-NI-koh-lah-oo test] microscopic examination of cells scraped from the vagina and cervix after staining with Papanicolaou stain; also called Pap test

papillary [PAP-ih-lar-ee] small, nipple-like, raised tissue

papilledema [PAP-il-eh-DEE-mah] inflammation and edema of the optic disc caused by increased intracranial pressure from a brain tumor or head trauma; also known as a choked disc

papule [pap-YOOL] a small, raised bump or skin lesion

para- [pair-ah] *prefix*; beside or outside

paracortex [pair-ah-KOR-teks] the area of the lymph node that is rich in T-cells

paradoxical breathing [pair-ah-DOX-ih-kal BREE-thing] acute respiratory distress in which the chest falls and the abdomen rises on inspiration

paralysis [pa-RAL-ih-sis] temporary or permanent loss of motor function that may be due to stroke, spinal cord injury, tumor, or other neurological disorder

paranasal sinuses [pair-ah-NAY-sal SIGH-nus-ez] sinus cavities located directly adjacent to the nasal passage

paranoia [pair-ah-NOY-ah] a symptom of a thought disorder characterized by persistent, fearful ideas about safety that are not based on reality

parasitic ovum [pair-ah-SIT-ik OH-vum] the eggs of organisms, such as worms, that live within a host

parasympathetic nervous system [PAR-ah-sym-pah-THET-ik NERV-us SIS-tem] part of the autonomic nervous system that includes nerve fibers originating in the cranial and sacral areas and terminating in glands and muscles; function is to slow the heart and stimulate peristalsis and vasodilation to conserve or restore body resources

parathyroid glands [pair-ah-THIGH-royd glanz] endocrine glands on the dorsal surfaces of the lateral lobes of the thyroid gland; secretes parathyroid hormone for calcium homeostasis in the blood

parathyroid hormone [pair-ah-THIGH-roid HOR-mohn] substance secreted by the parathyroid gland that regulates calcium and phosphorus metabolism

parathyroidectomy [pair-ah-thigh-royd-EK-toh-mee] surgical removal of one or more of the parathyroid glands

parenchyma [pair-EN-kih-mah] parts of an organ essential to its function rather than its physical structure

-paresis [pair-ee-sis] *suffix*; minor weakness or paralysis

paresthesia [pair-es-THE-zee-ah] abnormal sensation of numbness and tingling without objective cause

parietal lobe [pair-RY-eh-tal lohb] the portion of the cerebrum located on the lateral and medial surfaces and covered by the parietal bone

parietal pleura [pair-RY-eh-tal PLOOR-ah] one of the two pleural membranes lining the thoracic cavity

parotitis [par-oh-TYE-tis] inflammation of the parotid gland, commonly referred to as mumps

Parkinson facies [PAR-kin-sen fay-seez] expressionless, masklike facial feature associated with Parkinson's disease

Parkinson's disease [par-kin-SONZ dis-EEZ] condition of slowly progressive degeneration of an area of the substantia nigra causing a decreased amount of dopamine; characterized by tremors, rigidity of muscles, and bradykinesia

paronychia [par-oh-NIK-ee-ah] inflammation with pus at the nail edges

paroxysm [PAIR-ok-sizm] sudden, recurrent symptoms of a disease

partial seizure [PAR-shul SEE-zure] brain dysfunction involving only limited areas of the brain with localized symptoms

-partum [pahr-tum] *suffix*; childbirth

parturition [par-tyoo-RISH-shun] labor and delivery of a fetus

patch [PATCH] a nonelevated skin lesion larger than 1 cm in diameter

patella [pah-TEL-lah] the small, rounded bone situated at the front of the knee; also known as the kneecap

patellapexy [pah-tel-lah-PEK-see] surgical fixation of the kneecap

patellar reflex [pah-TEL-lar REE-fleks] striking the patellar ligaments resulting in extension of the lower leg

patency [PAY-ten-see] condition of having a wide, open lumen

patent ductus arteriosus [PAT-unt DUK-tus ar-TEER-ee-OH-sus] the ductus arteriosus remains open after birth, allowing oxygenated blood back into the lungs through the foramen oval; characterized by thrill, fremitus, and signs of congestive heart failure

pathogen [PATH-oh-jen] a microorganism capable of producing disease such as bacterium, virus, or fungus

pathogenesis [path-oh-JEN-eh-sis] an agent that is the causative agent of a disease; for example, bacteria

pathologic fracture [PATH-oh-LAW-jik FRAK-shur] displacement of a bone caused by a disease process such as osteoporosis, bone cancer, or metastases

-pathy [path-ee] *suffix*; a disease process

patient [PAY-shent] one who suffers from a medical condition requiring treatment by a clinician

patient-controlled analgesia (PCA) [PAY-shent-kon-TROLD an-al-JEE-zee-uh] a method for administering an intravenous narcotic agent, such as morphine, using a computerized pump that permits the patient to self-administer doses of medication within preset parameters

-pause [pawz] *suffix*; pause or cessation

peak expiratory flow [PEEK eks-PIH-ra-tor-ee flow] a measurement of the volume of air after forced expiration

pectoral girdle [PEK-toh-ral GIR-dl] muscles of the upper chest and shoulders

pectoralis major muscle [PEK-toh-ral-is MAY-jur MUS-sel] the large, triangular muscle of the chest that flexes the chest and internally rotates the humerus when contracted

pectoralis minor muscle [PEK-toh-ral-is MY-nor MUS-sel] muscle that moves the scapula against the thorax

pectus excavatum [PEK-tus eks-kah-VAH-tum] a congenital deformity of the bony thorax in which the sternum, particularly the xyphoid process, is bent inward, creating a hollow depression in the anterior chest; treatment is often surgery

pedicle [PED-ih-kl] a bony process that extends out the back of the body of vertebrae

pediculosis [ped-dik-yoo-LOH-sis] skin infection caused by lice infestation; denoted by the location: head (capitis), eyelashes (palpebrarum), body (corpus), or pubis

pedunculated polyp [peh-DUNG-kyoo-lay-ted PAW-lip] a fleshy abnormal growth in the intestine or other tissues characterized by a thin stalk supporting a ball-shaped, irregular top

pellagraphia [pel-lah-GRAF-ee-uh] repetition of phrases and words in writing, indicative of brain or psychiatric pathology

pelvic inflammatory disease (PID) [PEL-vik in FLAM-ah-tor-ee dis-EEZ] infection of the uterus, fallopian tubes, and adjoining structures caused by infectious agents spreading upward in the female reproductive tract, producing fever, chills, vaginal discharge, dysuria, and dyspareunia; common infectious agents are *Chlamydia trachomatis*, *Neisseria gonorrhea*, and *Escherichia coli*

pelvis [PEL-vis] a basin-shaped structure that includes the hip, sacrum, and coccyx of the spinal column; examples include the bony and renal pelvis

pemphigus [PEM-fi-gus] skin disorder with groups of bulla

-penia [peh-nee-ah] *suffix*; abnormal decline, deficiency

penis [PEE-nis] external genitalia of the male, composed of erectile tissue

pent- [pent] *prefix*; five

-pepsia [pep-see-uh] *suffix*; pertaining to digestion

pepsin [PEP-sin] a digestive enzyme from the stomach that breaks down food protein into large protein molecules

pepsinogen [pep-SYN-oh-jen] a precursor of pepsin that exists in granular form in the gastric glands

peptic ulcer [PEP-tik UL-sur] erosion of the upper gastrointestinal (GI) tract caused by excessive secretion of acid

peptidase [PEP-tih-days] digestive enzyme secreted by the small intestine that converts peptides to amino acids

per- [per] *prefix*; through or extremely

percussion [per-KUS-shun] tapping the finger of one hand, spread over a large body cavity to detect characteristics of underlying structures; use of a cupped hand to strike the chest and various lung fields in efforts to break up mucus for expectoration or suctioning

percutaneous [per-kyoo-TAY-nee-us] to go through the skin; used in reference to application of topical medication by friction or by insertion of a needle through the skin

percutaneous endoscopic gastrostomy (PEG) [per-kyoo-TAY-nee-us EN-doh-SKAW-pik gas-TRAWS-toh-mee] insertion of a permanent feeding tube through the abdominal wall using visual guidance from an endoscope passed through the mouth into the stomach

percutaneous lithoscopy [per-kyoo-TAY-nee-us LITH-oh-scop-ee] endoscope is inserted in a percutaneous approach into the kidney to remove a stone embedded in the renal pelvis or adjacent structures

percutaneous transluminal coronary angioplasty [per-kyoo-TAY-nee-us trans-LEW-mi-nul KOR-uh-nerr-ee AN-jee-oh-plas-tee] an invasive cardiac procedure in which a balloon catheter is used to restore blood flow in a blocked vessel

perfusion [per-FYOO-shun] passage of fluid and gases through vessels in an organ

perfusion deficit [per-FYOO-shun DEF-ih-sit] inadequate blood flow to tissue due to narrowing or occlusion

peri- [pair-ee] *prefix*; around

perianal [pair-ee-AYE-nal] anatomical region around the anus

pericardiocentesis [pair-ee-kahr-dee-oh-sen-TEE-sis] drainage of the pericardial sac by a needle or catheter

pericarditis [per-ee-kar-DYE-tis] inflammation of the heart muscle which may have bacterial, viral, fungal, autoimmune or other etiology. Key symptoms include an audible friction rub upon auscultation, fever, cough, and chest pain that worsens when lying down

pericardium [pair-ee-KAHR-dee-um] closed sac encircling the heart

periodontal membrane [per-ee-oh-DON-tal MEM-brayn] soft tissue that is immediately adjacent to the surface of a tooth and anchors it in place

perilymph [PER-ih-lymf] fluid found in the osseous labyrinth of the inner ear

perimetrium [per-ih-MEE-tree-um] outermost wall of the uterus

perimysium [per-ih-MIS-ee-um] the fibrous sheath that surrounds each bundle of skeletal muscle fibers

perineal prostatectomy [per-ih-NEE-al praw-stay-TEK-toh-mee] surgical excision of the prostate gland through the perineum

perineorrhaphy [per-ih-nee-OR-af-ee] suturing of the perineum, often due to a tear sustained during vaginal delivery of a fetus

perineurium [per-ih-NEW-ree-um] connective tissue around a bundle of nerve fibers

periosteum [PAIR-ee-AWS-tee-um] a thick, fibrous membrane that covers the outer surface of a bone

peripheral nervous system [peh-RIF-eh-tal NER-vus SIS-tem] nerves and ganglia outside the brain and spinal cord

peripheral vascular disease [peh-RIF-eh-tal VAS-kew-lur dis-EEZ] circulatory disorder characterized by limited or occluded small arteries and arterioles supplying the extremities

peristalsis [pair-ih-STAL-sis] the movement of food through the intestine via smooth-muscle contraction

peritoneal cavity [pair-ih-toh-NEE-al KAV-ih-tee] the space between the parietal and visceral layers of the peritoneum, used in peritoneal dialysis

peritoneal dialysis [pair-ih-toh-NEE-al dye-AL-ih-sis] filtration procedure that administers a dialysis solution in the peritoneal cavity to filter blood, correct electrolyte imbalances, and remove toxins, wastes, and drugs from the body

peritoneum [per-ih-toh-NEE-um] connective tissue that lines the abdominal cavity

peritonitis [pair-ih-toh-NIGH-tis] inflammation and infection of the peritoneum; this occurs when an ulcer, diverticulum, or cancerous tumor penetrates into the abdominopelvic cavity

peritonsillar [pair-ee-TAWN-sih-lar] tissue of the throat immediately adjacent to tonsils

periumbilical [pair-ee-uhm-BIL-ik-ul] abdominal area around or above the umbilicus

pernicious [per-NISH-us] a harmful, destructive, or fatal condition

peroneal [peh-roh-NEE-al] pertaining to the muscles over the fibula

peroneus longus muscle [peh-roh-NEE-us LON-gus MUS-sel] muscle of the anterior surface of the lower leg that extends the foot when contracted

pertussis [per-TUS-is] whooping cough, an infectious disease with characteristic "whoop" sound during coughing

petechia [pee-TEE-kee-ah] spot of hemorrhaging

petechiae [peh-TEE-kee-aye] pinpoint hemorrhages on the skin occurring due to platelet deficiency

-pexy [pek-see] *suffix*; suspension or fixation by surgical intervention

Peyer's patches [PY-erz PACH-ez] multiple lymphoid follicles in a compact space that form the elevations of the mucous membrane of the small intestine

phacoemulsification [FAY-koh-ee-MUL-sih-fih-KAY-shun] small, self-sealing incision made in the cornea, followed by an ultrasonic probe insertion to deliver sound waves to break up the lens; pieces of the lens are removed with irrigation and aspiration

phagocyte [FAY-goh-site] white blood cell that engulfs and digests foreign debris or particles

phagocytic crust [FAY-goh-sit-ik krust] cells found within the lungs that engulf debris and foreign compounds

phagocytosis [fay-goh-sigh-TOE-sis] the engulfing and ingesting of bacteria and old cells

phalangeal ray [fah-LAN-jee-al RAY] fingers in a spread-out fashion

phalanges [fah-LAN-jeez] bones of the fingers and toes

pharyngeal [fair-IN-jee-al] pertaining to the throat

pharyngocele [fair-IN-goh-seal] swelling or herniation of the pharynx

pharyngospasm [fair-IN-goh-spazm] involuntary contraction or spasm of the pharynx

pharynx [FAIR-inks] throat; structure through which air passes during inhalation and exhalation

phenylalanine hydroxylose [fen-il-AL-ah-neen hy-DROX-ee-los] an enzyme necessary to break down phenylalanine hydroxylase into tyrosine; lack of this enzyme results in excess phenylalanine in the blood that eventually spills over into the urine

phenylketonuria [fen-il-kee-toh-NYOO-ree-uh] a congenital disorder resulting in the inability to metabolize the amino acid phenylalanine due to the deficiency of the enzyme phenylalanine hydroxylase, causing severe neurological, skin, and psychiatric disorders; treatment consists of dietary restriction of phenylalanine

pheochromocytoma [fee-oh-KRO-moh-sy-TOH-ma] a tumor of functional chromaffin cells of the adrenal medulla that produces excess catecholamines, causing hypertension, nausea, headache, anxiety, and dyspnea

-phil [fill] *suffix*; attraction to

-philia [fill-ee-ah] *suffix*; attraction to

philtrum [FIL-trum] vertical groove in the skin of the upper lip**phimosis** [fih-MOH-sis] tightened foreskin

phimosis [fih-MOH-sis] tightened foreskin that cannot be retracted

phlebitis [flee-BYE-tis] vein inflammation

phlebo- [fleb-oh] *prefix*; vein

phlebosclerosis [FLEB-oh-skle-ROH-sis] hardening of the veins

phlebostenosis [FLEB-oh-sten-OH-sis] constriction or narrowing of a vein

phlebothrombosis [fleb-oh-throm-BOH-sis] formation of a clot in a vein resulting from inflammation

phlebotomy [fleh-BOHT-oh-mee] medical procedure of drawing a sample of venous blood into a vacuum tube

phlegm [FLEM] viscous, stringy mucus secreted by the walls of the respiratory tract

phobia [FOH-bee-ah] intense, unreasonable fear of a specific object or situation

-phobia [foh-bee-ah] *suffix*; pertaining to extreme fear

phocomelia [foh-ko-MEE-lee-ah] congenital malformation where hands and/or feet are directly attached to the trunk; sometimes due to prenatal exposure to thalidomide

phono- [foh-noh] *prefix*; voice, sound

phorometry [foh-RAWM-eh-tree] medical procedure to select the strength of lens that corrects the patient's refractive error and provides 20/20 vision

photo- [foe-toh] *prefix*; light

photoablation [foh-toh-ab-LAY-shun] use of a laser light to destroy or cut tissue

photophobia [foh-toh-FOH-bee-ah] intolerance to light

photoreceptors [FOH-toh-ree-SEP-torz] specialized light-sensitive cells of the eye such as rods and cones

photorefractive keratotomy (PRK) [foh-toh-ree-FRAK-tiv ker-ah-TOT-oh-mee] use of an excimer laser to reshape the curvature of the cornea without the creation of a corneal surface flap

photoretinitis [foh-toh-ret-ih-NY-tis] inflammation of the retina due to prolonged exposure to intense light

phrenic [FREN-ik] pertaining to the diaphragm

phrenic nerve [FREN-ik NERV] nerve that stimulates the diaphragm to contract, thereby initiating respiration

phrenoplegia [fren-oh-PLEE-jee-uh] paralysis of the diaphram

phrenospasm [FREN-oh-spazm] involuntary spasm or twitching of the diaphragm

-phylaxis [fil-ak-sis] *suffix*; protection or preventative measure

physical therapy [FIZ-ih-kal THAIR-ah-pee] medical interventions using active or passive exercises to improve a patient's range of motion, joint mobility, muscular strength, and balance

physiologic anorexia [fiz-ee-oh-LOJ-ik an-oh-REK-see-ah] decrease in appetite due to physical illness

physiology [fiz-ee-AWL-oh-jee] study of the function of the body

-physis [fih-sis] *suffix*; to grow

pia mater [PEE-ah MAY-ter] the vascular and innermost of the three meninges covering the brain and spinal cord

pica [PY-ka] eating disorder characterized by craving of nonfood items such as clay, paste, or coffee grounds

pilonidal cyst [py-loh-NY-dal SYST] hair that has been encapsulated in a dermal cyst

pilosebaceous melanin [pye-loh-se-BAY-shus MEL-ah-nin] black or dark brown pigment produced by cells called melanocytes

pineal gland [PYE-nee-al gland] a pinecone–shaped organ in the brain that secretes melatonin; also known as pineal body

pinna [PIN-nah] external structure of the ear

pinocytosis [PIN-oh-sy-TOH-sis] a process wherein a cell engulfs liquid by encircling the substance, forming fluid-filled vesicles

pisiform [PIS-ah-form] a small, pea-sized bone located in the wrist

pituitary dwarfism [pi-TEW-ih-tear-ee DWORF-iz-um] grossly decreased physical height; disproportion among bodily parts due to inadequate growth hormone levels

pituitary gigantism [pi-TEW-ih-tear-ee jye-GAN-tiz-um] excessive growth caused by hypersecretion of pituitary growth hormone, commonly due to pituitary adenoma

pituitary gland [pi-TEW-ih-tear-ee gland] hypophysis; so-called "master gland" that orchestrates endocrine function

pivot joint [PIV-ot joynt] a synovial joint in which movement is limited to rotation

placebo [pla-SEE-boh] an inactive substance administered in controlled research studies; when the power of suggestion is used to trigger a belief in and response to medication

placenta [pla-SEN-tah] the organ of fetomaternal circulatory exchange that is attached to the uterine mucosa

-plagia [PLAY-gee-ah] *suffix*; paralysis

-plakia [play-kee-uh] *suffix*; condition of forming hard deposits or plaque

planovagus [PLAY-no-VAY-gus] flat or flaccid longitudinal arch of the foot

plantar fasciitis [PLAN-tar fas-ee-EYE-tis] inflammation of the fascia in the arch of the foot, with the greatest pain at the calcaneal attachment

plantar flexion [PLAN-tar FLEK-shun] movement of the foot and ankle such that the toes point downward

plantar grasp reflex [PLAN-tar grasp REE-fleks] an automatic neurological response to stimulation of the foot that results in a curling movement as if gripping the finger; found in newborns up to eight months

plantar reflex [PLAN-tar REE-fleks] flexion of the foot and toes when the bottom surface of the foot is stimulated

plantar wart [PLAN-tar wart] viral lesion on the foot

plaque [PLAK] lipid deposition on the arterial wall of a vessel or structure

-plasia [play-zee-ah] *suffix*; growth

-plasm [pla-zim] *suffix*; cell or tissue substance

plasma cells [PLAZ-muh sellz] antibody-producing cells derived from B cells

plasmapheresis [PLAZ-muh-fer-EE-sis] procedure in which plasma is separated from the blood cells by rapid spinning in a centrifuge; the blood cells are returned to the donor

plasminogen [plaz-MIN-oh-gen] drugs that dissolve already-formed blood clots by converting plasminogen to an enzyme that breaks the fibrin strands

-plasty [plas-tee] *suffix*; surgical reconstruction or repair

play therapy [PLAY THAIR-ah-pee] use of toys and other objects to help young children express emotions or to reenact traumatic or abusive events under the guidance of a mental health professional

pleura [PLUR-uh] outermost membrane of the lung

pleural effusion [PLUR-al ee-FYOO-shun] any abnormal collection of fluid in the pleural cavity

pleuralgia [plur-AL-jee-ah] pain originating in the lining of the lung or the chest wall; also called intercostal neuralgia

pleurisy [PLUR-ih-see] inflammation of the pleura due to infection or trauma; also called pleuritis

pleurodynia [PLU-roh-dih-nee-ah] pain arising from inflammation or infection of the lung

plexus [PLEK-sus] a network of nerves, blood vessels, or lymphatic vessels throughout the body

plica [PLY-kah] one of the smooth folds of the synovial membrane of the joint capsule of the knee

-pnea [nee-ah] *suffix*; breathing

pneumocentesis [noo-MOH-sen-TEE-sis] surgical puncture of a lung for the purpose of removing abnormal collection of fluid

pneumoconiosis [new-moh-ko-nee-OH-sis] progressive lung disease caused by prolonged exposure to metallic or mineral dusts, frequently seen as an occupational exposure; symptoms include progressive lung irritation, cough, dyspnea, malaise, and frequent respiratory infections

Pneumocystis carinii [NOO-moh-SIS-tis kah-REE-nee-eye] an infectious microorganism that causes inflammation of the lung, formation of granulomas, and fibrosis in the bronchioles and alveoli; often associated with immunosuppressive disorders

pneumonectomy [NOO-mon-NEK-toh-mee] surgical removal of an entire lung, usually performed to treat lung cancer

pneumonia [noo-MOH-nee-ah] infection of lung; may be from bacterial or viral sources

pneumonic plague [nyoo-MON-ik playg] a fast-moving, often fatal infection characterized by areas of pulmonary consolidation, fevers, pain, and bloody sputum

pneumotaxic [new-moh-TAK-sic] area of brain that regulates or controls the respiratory rate

pneumothorax [noo-moh-THOR-aks] collection of air in the pleural cavity which may result in partial or complete collapse of the lung

-poiesis [po-ee-sis] *suffix*; to form or produce

poliomyelitis [POL-ee-oh-mi-LIH-tis] inflammation of the gray matter of the brain caused by a virus, often resulting in spinal and muscle deformity and paralysis

poly- [pawl-ee] *prefix*; many

polyadenoma [POL-ee-ah-den-OH-mah] malignant tumor involving many glands throughout the body

polycystic kidney disease [pol-ee-SIS-tik KID-nee dis-EEZ] an inherited disorder characterized by deformed nephrons that develop multiple grapelike cysts throughout the kidneys; requires dialysis and kidney transplant

polycythemia [POL-ee-sy-THEE-mee-uh] condition of increased numbers of red cells in the blood to increase the amount of hemoglobin available to carry oxygen

polycythemia vera [POL-ee-sy-THEE-mee-uh VER-ah] a chronic disorder of excessive production of red blood cells and hemoglobin concentration

polydactyly [PAWL-ee-DAK-tih-lee] congenital condition of having extra fingers or toes

polydipsia [PAWL-ee-DIP-see-ah] excessive thirst, often associated with diabetes

polykaryocyte [pol-ee-KAR-ee-oh-syt] cells with more than one nuclei

polymyositis [pawl-ee-migh-oh-SIGH-tis] autoimmune disease characterized by muscle inflammation and atrophy

polyneuritis [pawl-ee-nu-RIGH-tis] inflammation involving two or more nerves; often due to nutritional deficits, especially of thiamine

polyp [PAW-lip] small, fleshy, benign or precancerous growth that arises from the mucosa; often found in the colon and sinuses

polypectomy [PAWL-ih-PEK-toh-mee] surgical removal of soft, pendulous tissues from the intestine, nasal cavity, sinuses, or vocal cords

polypeptide [pol-ee-PEP-tyd] a substance composed of two or more amino acids

polyphagia [pawl-ee-FAY-jee-ah] excessive intake of food which can be due to hyperthyroidism, diabetes mellitus, or a psychiatric illness

polypharmacy [pol-ee-FAR-mah-see] concurrent use of multiple drugs, both with and without the knowledge of the medical team, giving rise to increased risk for drug to drug interaction

polythelia [pol-ee-THE-lee-uh] condition of having more than one nipple on a breast

polyuria [pawl-ee-YOO-ree-ah] excessive urination

pons [PONZ] brain tissue between the medulla and midbrain; metencephalon

popliteal artery [pop-LIT-ee-al AR-ter-ee] blood vessel that delivers oxygenated blood to the area of the knee and calf

popliteal pulse [pop-LIT-ee-al puls] a palpable throbbing movement detected at the dorsal-medial surface of the knee

popliteus muscle [pop-LIT-ee-us MUS-sel] muscle located behind the knee joint that flexes and assists in rotation of the thigh when flexed

pore [POR] a very small opening on the surface of the epithelium

portal hepatis [POR-tal HE-pa-tis] anatomic landmark on the liver where the portal vein, hepatic artery, hepatic ducts, and hepatic lymphatic vessels enter at the point of the transverse fissure that separates the caudate and quadrate lobes

positive pressure ventilation [POZ-ih-tiv PRESH-ur ven-ti-LAY-shun] a method of mechanically assisted breathing that keeps the airway open by maintaining pressure within the airway that is higher than the body surface pressure

positron emission tomography (PET) [POZ-ih-tron ee-MISH-shun toh-MOG-rah-fee] a diagnostic study employing computer analysis of photons detected to determine localization of metabolic and physiologic function

post- [pohst] *prefix*; behind or after

post-synaptic membrane [post-sin-AP-tik MEM-brayn] the membrane of a neuron immediately beyond the synapse

post-synaptic receptors [post-sin-AP-tik ree-CEP-tors] neuroreceptors located adjacent to the synapse

posterior [pohs-TEER-ee-or] back

posterior chamber [pos-TEER-ee-or CHAM-ber] thin space behind the iris

posterior column [pos-TEER-ee-or KOL-uhm] portion of white matter located bilaterally on the posterior surface of the spinal cord

posterior fornix [pos-TEER-ee-or FOR-niks] the deepest of the four recesses of the cervix

posterior inferior vena cava [pos-TEER-ee-or in-FEER-ee-or vee-nah kay-vuh] the primary vein that drains blood from the lower portion of the body and joins the two common iliac veins and ends at the right atrium of the heart

posterior parathyroid [pos-TEER-ee-or pair-uh-THIGH-royd] endocrine gland which regulates blood calcium and phosphorus ion levels by excretion of parathyroid hormone

posteroanterior [POS-tee-roh-an-TER-ree-or] literal meaning is "from back to front"; radiological use of term indicates passage of x-rays from back to front

postganglionic nerve fiber [POST-gang-lee-AWN-ik nerv FY-ber] an axon of the sympathetic and parasympathetic neuron located after the ganglionic terminus at the muscle or gland

postictal period [post-IK-tal PEER-ee-od] time frame following seizure activity during which the level of consciousness is decreased

postmortem examination [post-MOHR-tum eks-am-ih-NAY-shun] inspection of the body after death to ascertain cause of death

postnatal [post-NAY-tal] period of life right after birth

postprandial [post-PRAN-dee-ul] after a meal

post-traumatic stress disorder (PTSD) [POST-tra-MAT-ik STRES dis-OR-der] ongoing disabling reaction to a traumatic situation or event, with numbed emotional response, disinterest in people and current events, and repeated reliving of the traumatic event; symptoms include chronic anxiety, insomnia, irritability, and occasional violent outbursts; previously known as combat fatigue or shell shock

postural drainage [POS-tur-al DRAYN-ij] positioning of the body to allow for removal of mucus from the airway such that it is facilitated by the forces of gravity; often accompanied by percussion to break secretions loose

pouch of Douglas [POWCH uv DUG-las] the rectouterine pouch at the base of the pelvis and behind the cervix

-prandial [pran-dee-al] *suffix*; meal

precancerous [pree-KAN-ser-us] benign tissue that has potential to become malignant

precapillary sphincters [pree-KAP-ih-lair-ee SFINK-terz] structures between capillaries and arterioles that regulate blood flow to capillaries

precocious puberty [pree-KOH-shus PEW-ber-tee] reaching physical maturity at an abnormally early age

premature atrial contractions [pree-mah-TCHUR AYE-tree-al kon-TRAK-shuns] early cardiac beats arising from the atrium of the heart due to early depolarization of the atrium; pathology may result from ischemic or enlarged myocardium or stress, nicotine, or caffeine

premenstrual dysphoric disorder (PMDD) [pree-MEN-stroo-al dis-FOR-ik dis-OR-der] depressive disorder associated with the period immediately prior to the onset of the menstrual cycle, including symptoms of premenstrual syndrome (PMS) (breast, joint, and muscle pains) with depression, anxiety, tearfulness, difficulty concentrating, and sleep and eating disturbances

prepuce [PREE-poos] foreskin of the penis, or the skin fold around the clitoris

presby- [prez-bee] *prefix*; old or age-related

presbycusis [pres-beh-KYOO-sis] decreased hearing associated with old age

presbyopia [pres-bee-OH-pee-ah] loss of ability to see near objects due to aging of the lens of the eye

pre-synaptic membrane [pre-syn-AP-tik MEM-brayn] surface of an axon that is before the synapse

priapism [PRI-ah-pizm] sustained, painful erection of the penis from a pathological state

primary follicle [PRY-mair-ee FOL-lih-kul] structure of the ovary consisting of an immature ovum and a single layer of epithelial cells

primary malnutrition [PRY-mair-ee mal-new-TRI-shun] ill health that originates from lack of ability to benefit from a normally healthy diet

pro- [proh] *prefix*; before

process [PRAW-sess] prominence or projection of tissue

procidentia [proh-sih-DEN-shah] third-degree prolapse of the uterus and cervix, extending through the introitus

proctocolitis [PROK-toh-koh-LY-tis] inflammation of the rectum and colon

prodrome [pro-DROM] symptoms indicative of approaching disease

progesterone [proh-JES-ter-ohn] a steroid hormone produced by the corpus luteum that produces changes in the endometrium in preparation for implantation of a fertilized egg

prognathism [PROG-nath-iz-im] abnormal facial configuration in which one or both of the jaws project forward

prognosis [prawg-NOH-sis] predicted outcome of a disease based upon the patient's condition and the usual progression of a disease

progressive supranuclear palsy (PSP) [prow-GRES-iv SOO-prah-nyoo-klee-ar PAWL-zee] a progressive neurological disorder characterized by neurodegenerative changes of the basal ganglia and the brain stem; symptoms include balance difficulties, sudden falls, rigidity, bradykinesia, myoclonus, slurred speech, swallowing difficulties, and impaired ability to perform voluntary eye movements

prolactin [pro-LAK-tin] hormone produced by the anterior pituitary gland that stimulates breast development and lactation during pregnancy

pronation [proh-NAY-shun] turning of the hand or other body part downward

pronator teres muscle [proh-NAY-tur TEER-eez MUS-sel] muscle that functions to produce medial arm rotation

prone [PROHN] positioning of the body lying down, facing downward

prophylaxis [pro-fil-AK-sis] any measure or action taken to prevent disease

proprioceptor [proh-pree-oh-SEP-tor] a nerve cell that senses change in position or location of body parts

prostate [PRAWS-tayt] a round gland surrounding the neck of the bladder and urethra, producing fluid that becomes part of semen

prostatectomy [pros-tay-TEK-toh-mee] surgical excision of all or portions of the prostate gland, often by a perineal incision

prostatic [proh-STAT-ik] pertaining to the prostate gland

prosthesis [pros-THEE-sis] any medical device that replaces a bodily part or function, such as an artificial leg after an amputation

protease [PRO-tee-ayse] class of enzymes that breaks down protein

protease inhibitor drug [PROH-tee-ayse in-HIB-ih-tor druhg] one of a class of medications used to treat human immunodeficiency virus by inhibiting the ability of the virus to replicate

proteinuria [proh-tee-NEW-ree-ah] abnormal presence of protein in the urine

prothrombin [proh-THRAWM-bin] a plasma coagulation factor (factor II) synthesized in the liver

proximal [PRAWK-sih-mal] near the center or point of origin

proximal flexor muscle [PRAWK-sih-mal FLEKS-or MUS-sel] a muscle that flexes a joint

pruritus [prew-RYE-tus] itching

pseud- [sood] *prefix*; false

pseudocyesis [SOO-doh-sy-EE-sis] psychiatric condition where the patient has signs and symptoms of pregnancy including lack of menses, morning sickness, and weight gain, but is not actually pregnant

pseudocyst [SOO-doh-sist] a formation that appears to be a cyst but lacks the internal fluid-filled nature of an actual cyst

pseudohypertrophy [SOO-doh-HY-per-troh-fee] enlargement of muscles due to infiltration by fatty tissue

pseudomembrane [soo-doh-MEM-brayn] a substance that is a false layer that resembles a membrane, often occurring in the respiratory tract, making breathing difficult

pseudophakia [soo-doh-FAY-kee-uh] condition where the lens of the eye is replaced with connective tissue

psoas muscle [SOH-as MUS-sel] muscle of the internal aspect of the hip that extends from the lumbar vertebrae to the lesser trochanter of the femur; contracture causes flexion and lateral movement of the spine

psoitis [soh-EYE-tis] inflammation and pain in the loins originating from the psoas muscle

psomophagia [soh-moh-FAY-jee-ah] habitually swallowing of food without completely chewing

psorelcosis [soh-rel-KOH-sis] ulcerative skin lesions occurring as a result of scabies

psoriasis [soh-RYE-ah-sis] autoimmune skin disease characterized by white, scaly plaques

psychiatrist [sigh-KY-ah-trist] a physician practicing in the specialty of mental health, diagnosing and treating patients with mental illness; subspecialties include child and adolescent, geriatric, psychosomatic medicine, addiction, and forensic

psychoanalysis [SIGH-koh-ah-NAL-ih-sis] the oldest school of psychotherapy, developed by Sigmund Freud, in which the ideas of conscious and subconscious experiences are analyzed in a lengthy process to facilitate reintegration and development of insight

psychologist [sigh-KAWL-oh-jist] mental health clinician who has a doctoral degree (PhD) in psychology and provides diagnostic testing and therapy sessions for individuals and groups in psychiatric hospitals, outpatient clinics, and schools

psychotherapy [sigh-koh-THAIR-ah-pee] any therapy facilitated by a mental health professional which uses verbal or nonverbal communication between a patient or a group to treat a mental disorder

psychrotherapy [sigh-kro-THER-ah-pee] use of cold temperature to treat a disease; used in removal of skin lesions such as warts

pterygium fiberousis [ter IJ-ee-um} a condition where the conjunctiva tissue extends across the cornea of the eye

ptilosis [tye-LOH-sis] loss of eyelashes due to disease or chemotherapy

ptosis [TOE-sis] drooping, downward placement of an organ or tissue

ptyalism [TYE-ah-lizm] excessive secretion of saliva; hypersalivation

ptyalith [TYE-ah-lith] a stone formed in the salivary gland

ptyalocele [tye-AL-oh-seel] a cyst formed in the salivary gland

ptyalogogue [tye-AL-oh-gog] pharmacological agent that causes an increase in the production of saliva

-ptysis [tye-sis] *suffix*; splitting

puberty [PYOO-ber-tee] development of genital maturity and of secondary sex characteristics, culminating in sexual maturity and ability to reproduce

pudendal [pyoo-DEN-dal] pertaining to female external genitalia

puerile [PYOO-eh-ril] concerning a child; childlike quality; used to describe lack of normal neurological or psychological functioning

pulmonary [PUL-moh-nair-ee] pertaining to the lungs, breathing

pulmonary artery [PUL-moh-nair-ee AR-ter-ee] vessel that carries deoxygenated blood from the right ventricle of the heart to the lungs for oxygenation

pulmonary atresia [PUL-moh-nair-ee ah-TREE-zee-ah] absence of the tricuspid or pulmonary valves

pulmonary circuit [PUL-moh-nair-ee SER-kut] circulation of the blood through the lungs via the pulmonary arteries and veins; transports unoxygenated blood from the right ventricle to the lungs, where the blood picks up oxygen, and then returns oxygenated blood from the lungs to the left atrium

pulmonary function test (PFT) [PUL-moh-nair-ee FUNK-shun test] a series of tests using diagnostic spirometry to determine lung capacities and volume

pulmonary perfusion scan [PUL-moh-nair-ee per-FYOO-shun skan] diagnostic study where the patient is given an injection of radioactive albumin into a vein to evaluate blood flow to the lungs using images produced by a gamma camera scanner

pulmonary semilunar valve [PUL-moh-nair-ee sem-ee-LEW-nur valv] valve between the heart and the pulmonary trunk

pulmonary veins [PUL-moh-nair-ee vaynz] vessels that carry oxygenated blood from the lungs to the heart

pulmonary ventilation scan [PUL-moh-nair-ee ven-tih-LAY-shun skan] diagnostic study where the patient inhales xenon gas and the images produced using a gamma camera denote the distribution of air in the lungs

pulmonic stenosis [pul-MOH-nik sten-OH-sis] narrowing of a valve that produces an obstruction of blood flow into the pulmonary artery, causing increased preload and right ventricular hypertrophy

pulmonologists [POL-moh-NAWL-oh-jists] physicians who practice in the treatment of respiratory conditions

pulse [PULS] a rhythmic expansion of the arterial wall in response to cardiac contraction

pulse oximeter [puls oks-IM-eh-ter] medical device used to measure the oxygen saturation in the tissue capillaries, using a cliplike device on the finger or earlobe

pulse oximetry [puls ok-SIM-eh-tree] measurement of the oxygen saturation of the blood

pulse points [PULS poyntz] specific anatomic locations where arterial pulsations are normally palpated, including the temporal, carotid, brachial, radial, ulnar, femoral, popliteal, posterior tibial, and dorsalis pedis

pulse pressure [puls PRESH-ur] difference between the systolic and diastolic blood pressure readings, which is normally ranges between 30 and 50 mm Hg

pulverize [PUL-ver-eyez] to reduce a hard substance to a fine powder consistency by mechanical means, often accomplished by ultrasound to break up calculi formed in the renal pelvis

punch biopsy [punch BY-op-see] removal of a circular piece of tissue for examination; usually performed on the cervix uteri

punch drunk syndrome [PUNCH drunk SIN-drom] neurological damage caused by multiple concussions resulting in functional presentation of abnormal gait and slowed movements

pupil [PYOO-pil] the dark center of the iris that allows light rays to enter the eye

pupillary reflex [PYOO-pil-air-ee REE-fleks] constriction of the iris of the eye due to stimulation with light

pupillary response [PYOO-pil-air-ee re-SPONS] assessment of the pupil's ability to constrict briskly and equally in response to a bright light

Purkinje fiber [per-KIN-jee FY-ber] cardiac muscle cell located beneath the endocardium and forming part of the electroconduction system of the heart

purpura [PUR-pur-ah] purple-colored, visible leakage of red blood cells into the subcutaneous tissue or mucous membranes; caused by a variety of mechanisms (trauma, clotting disorders, allergy)

pustules [PUS-toolz] skin elevations that contain pus

pyelitis [pye-eh-LYE-tis] inflammation of the kidney pelvis and calyces

pyelocaliectasis [PYE-ee-loh-KAL-ih-EK-tay-sis] dilation of the renal pelvis and renal calices

pyelonephritis [pye-eh-loh-ne-FRYE-tis] interstitial inflammation of the kidney

pylorostenosis [pye-LOR-oh-steh-NOH-sis] constriction or narrowing of the valve at the end of the stomach due to ulcer, disease, malignant tumor, or scarring and hypertrophy of the mucosa and submucosa

pylorus [pye-LOR-us] the valve at the terminus of the stomach that keeps food in the stomach, then opens to allow passage into the duodenum

pyoderma [pye-oh-DER-mah] any disease of the skin that produces pus

pyothorax [pye-oh-THOR-aks] pus in the pleural cavity, known as empyema

pyrexia [pye-REK-see-uh] increased temperature; fever

pyrogen [PYE-roh-jen] an agent, such as bacteria, viruses, or inflammatory disorders, that causes fever

pyrosis [pye-ROH-sis] temporary inflammation of the esophagus due to reflux of stomach acid

pyuria [pye-YOOR-ee-ah] presence of high numbers of white blood cells in the urine, often attributable to infection of the bladder and urethra

Q

QRS complex [Q-R-S KOM-pleks] section of the electrocardiogram (ECG) showing the duration of ventricular depolarization

quadrant [KWAH-drant] one of four parts; for example, abdominal quadrants

quadri- [kwad-rih] *prefix;* four

quadriceps muscles [KWAH-dri-seps MUS-selz] muscle group of the anterior thigh that extends the leg, composed of recta femoris, vastus intermedius, vastus lateralis, and vastus medialis

quadriplegia [kwad-ri-PLEE-jee-ah] paralysis of all four limbs caused by a spinal cord lesion

R

rachilysis [ray-KIL-ih-sis] treatment of spinal curvature using pressure and traction

rachiodynia [ray-kee-oh-DY-nee-uh] pain in the structures of the back

rachischisis [rah-KIS-kih-sis] congenital condition of a spinal fissure

rachitis [rah-KY-tis] inflammation of the spine

radial artery [RAY-dee-al AR-ter-ee] blood vessel that supplies oxygenated blood to the forearm and hand

radial pulse [RAY-dee-al puls] bounding, throbbing sensation at the distal portion of the radius of the forearm with each contraction of the heart

radiation therapy [ray-dee-AYE-shun THAIR-ah-pee] use of radioactive elements as diagnostic and therapeutic interventions

radical neck dissection [RAD-ih-kal nek dye-SEK-shun] a surgical procedure to treat extensive cancer of the mouth and neck; includes removing parts of the jawbone, tongue, larynx, lymph nodes, and muscles of the neck

radiculitis [rah-dik-yoo-LY-tis] inflammation of a nerve root characterized by pain and hypersensitivity

radioactive iodine uptake test [ray-dee-oh-AK-tiv EYE-oh-dyne UP-tayk test] examination used to determine the rate of radioiodine absorption in the thyroid

radioallergosorbent test (RAST) [RAY-dee-oh-AL-er-goh-SOR-bent test] a blood test in which radioimmunoassay is used to measure the presence of IgE antibodies in the blood to detect allergies to various substances, such as certain cosmetics, animal fur, dust, and grasses

radiocarpal joint [RAY-dee-oh-KAR-pal joynt] the articular surface that joins the head of the radius and the bones of the wrist

radiofrequency rhizotomy [RAY-dee-oh-FREE-qwen-see ry-ZOH-toh-mee] procedure to relieve pain in the trigeminal nerve by use of radio waves through the skin

radiography [RAY-dee-oh-graf-ee] production of a shadow-type image on photographic film by exposure of film to x-rays

radioimmunoassay [RAY-dee-oh-im-yoo-noh-as-say] study of antigens, antibodies, enzymes, and hormones using radiolabeled reactants

radioiodine [ray-dee-oh-EYE-oh-dine] radioactive isotope of iodine

radionuclide scan [ray-dee-oh-NEW-klide skan] computer-generated images made by isolating radionuclides in the bloodstream for diagnostic purposes

radiopharmaceutical [RAY-dee-oh-farm-ah-sue-tic-ahl] drug containing a radioactive substance that travels to a specific body region or organ that will be scanned (i.e., CAT scan)

radius [RAY-dee-us] bone of the lateral forearm that is aligned with the thumb

ramus [RAY-mus] a branching structure from a larger anatomical structure such as a nerve or blood vessel

Ranvier's node [ron-vee-AYZ nohd] the nonmylenated segment of the neuron

Raynaud's disease [ray-NOZ dis-EEZ] a disorder characterized by numbness in fingers or toes due to intermittent constriction of arterioles

re- [ree] *prefix*; back or again

rebound tenderness [REE-bownd TEN-der-ness] reflexive, sharp pain induced by sudden release of fingers on the abdomen; indicative of peritonitis or appendicitis

receptor [ree-SEP-tor] a sensory nerve ending that receives a chemical message by linking or binding to a specific factor, drug, hormone, antigen, or neurotransmitter

recession [ree-SESH-un] the moving back or shortening of, for example, a muscle

recovery position [ree-KUV-er-ee po-ZIH-shun] posture used to encourage full lung expansion where the patient is placed on the left side, with the left arm extended by the left ear and the right leg crossed over the left leg

rectocele [REK-toh-seel] protrusion of the wall of the rectum that pushes on the adjacent wall of the vagina, causing it to collapse and partially block the vaginal canal

rectoscope [REK-toh-skohp] instrument used to visualize the rectum

rectouterine pouch [rek-toh-YOO-ter-een powch] a pocket in the abdominal pelvic cavity at the lowest gravitational point where fluids and bacteria tend to collect; also known as the pouch of Douglas

rectum [REK-tum] a short, straight segment of bowel connecting the sigmoid colon to the outside of the body

rectus abdominus muscles [REK-tus ab-DOM-ih-nus MUS-selz] paired muscles of the abdomen extending the entire length of the vertical structure of the abdomen, functioning to compress the abdominal contents

rectus femoris muscle [REK-tus FEM-o-ris MUS-sel] muscle of the posterior thigh

red blood cells [RED BLUD sellz] mature erythrocytes that contain hemoglobin

reducible hernia [re-DEW-si-bul HUR-nee-ah] abnormal protrusion of an organ through a wall or cavity that can be physically manipulated back into normal position

referred pain [ree-FERD payn] discomfort that is felt in a different location than where it originates

reflex [REE-fleks] an involuntary movement or action due to a particular stimulus

reflex apnea [REE-fleks AP-nee-uh] to gasp; sudden or temporary loss of breath

reflux [REE-fluks] abnormal backward flow of fluid

refractory [ree-FRAK-tor-ee] unable to be resolved by treatment

refractory hypoxemia [ree-FRAK-tor-ee hy-pok-SEE-mee-ah] lack of normal amount of oxygen in the blood that does not respond to oxygen therapy or medications

reframing [ree-FRAYM-ing] therapeutic communication technique that focuses on changing the emotional perspective from which an experience is interpreted

registration [rej-is-TRAY-shun] memory encoding or learning in the central nervous system

regression [rih-GRESH shun] to move backward to a previous state of events, previous development, or primitive behavior

regurgitation [ree-GUR-jih-TAY-shun] the reflux of small amounts of food and acid back into the mouth

rehabilitation [REE-hab-il-it-TAY-shun] restoration of an individual to the highest level possible following an injury, functional loss, addiction, or incarceration

relapse [REE-laps] recurrence of a disease after a period of remission or recovery

reminiscence therapy [rem-in-is-ANS THAIR-ah-pee] psychotherapeutic technique that encourages individuals to review past pleasant experiences as a means of restoring self-esteem and personal satisfaction; this is used particularly with older adult clients

remission [ree-MISH-un] a period of time when symptoms of a disease are absent or greatly diminished

renal artery [REE-nal AR-ter-ee] paired blood vessels of the kidneys that supply oxygenated blood to the kidneys, suprarenal glands, and ureters

renal calculi [REE-nal KAL-kew-lye] kidney stones

renal capsule [REE-nal cap-sul] tissue attached immediately around the kidney and comprised of two layers: fibrous renal capsule and adipose renal capsule

renal carcinoma [REE nal kahr-si-NOH-muh] cancerous tumor of the kidney

renal colic [REE-nal KAWL-ik] sudden, severe, sharp pain originating from the area of the back over the kidney, associated with spasms, due to presence of an embedded renal stone

renal failure [REE-nal FAIL-yer] malfunctioning kidneys such that they are unable to excrete wastes, concentrate urine, and conserve electrolytes; may be characterized as acute or chronic

renal hypertension [REE-nal high-pur-TEN-shun] elevation of blood pressure due to renal artery atherosclerosis or other kidney diseases

renal hypoplasia [REE-nal high-poh-PLAY-zee-ah] a kidney of small size but with normal function except that it contains nephrons of smaller size or fewer number

renal ptosis [REE-nal TOH-sis] kidney drop resulting from loss of supporting adipose tissue

renal pyramid [REE-nal PEER-ah-mid] the cone-shaped structures forming the kidney medulla

renal transplantation [REE-nal TRANS-plan-tay-shun] the process of placing a donor kidney into a patient

renal vein [REE-nal vayn] paired blood vessels of the kidneys that return deoxygenated blood from the kidneys, suprarenal glands, and ureters

renin [REE-nin] enzyme released by the juxtaglomerular cells when there is a drop in renal blood flow that converts angiotensin to constrict blood vessels and maintain blood pressure

replication [rep-lih-KAY-shun] making an identical duplicate of DNA during the early stages of mitosis or meiosis

repression [ree-PRESH-hun] an unconscious defense mechanism that pushes painful, traumatic events, anxiety, or guilt-producing knowledge into the sub-conscious, where it is dormant but able to resurface

resection [ree-SEK-shun] to cut out and remove

residual volume [REE-zid-u-AWL VOL-yoom] the volume of air that remains in the lungs at all times; average = 1,500 cc

resocialization [ree-sosh-al-eye-ZAY-shun] supportive measures to reintegrate a client into family and community life following a critical or long-term hospitalization

resorption [ree-SORP-shun] to remove by the process of absorption

respiration [res-pir-AYE-shun] the process of exchanging oxygen and carbon dioxide in the body; breathing movements

respiratory center [RES-pi-ra-tor-ee SEN-ter] a group of nerve cells in the pons and medulla that control breathing

resting potential [RES-ting poh-TEN-shul] base condition of the nerve due to unequal distribution of ions inside and outside the cell, typically –70 millivolts (mV)

restless leg syndrome [REST-less leg SIN-drom] condition of unknown etiology where the patient has the urge to move the legs to such a degree that it prevents rest and/or sleep

restraint [ree-STRAYNT] any method of restricting movement with cloth, belts, and other devices to prevent harm to the patient and others

retained placenta [re-TAYND pla-SEN-tah] failure to deliver the placenta within 30 minutes after childbirth

retardation [ree-tar-DAY-shun] slowed or incomplete development or function

retention [ree-TEN-shun] ability to recall; inability to defecate, urinate, or expel other bodily substances normally

reticuloendothelial system [ree-TIK-yoo-loh-en-doh-THEE-lee-ul SIS tem] the collective, coordinated action of phagocytes in the liver, lungs, lymph nodes, and spleen that engulfs foreign substances in the body

retina [RET ih-nah] membrane lining the posterior cavity of the eye that contains rods and cones

retinaculum [RET-ih-NAK-yoo-lum] nearly translucent band of fibrous tissue and fascia that holds the extensor and flexor tendons that cross the wrist and ankle

retinal detachment [RET-ih-nal dee-TACH-ment] separation of the retina from the choroid layer of the eye due to trauma, aging, or diabetes causing the blood vessels to become increasingly fragile

retinitis pigmentosa [RET-ih-NY-tis pig-men-TOH-sah] abnormal deposits of pigmentation behind the rods and cones, causing loss of color or night, central, or peripheral vision that may progress to blindness

retinopathy [ret-ih-NOP-ah-thee] any disorder that causes destruction or disruption of the function of the retina

retinopexy [RET-ih-noh-PEK-see] surgical procedure used to re-attach a detached retina using cryotherapy to freeze the tissue and fix all three layers (sclera, choroid, retina) together

retinoschisis [ret-ih-NOS-kih-sis] a split or tear in the retina of the eye

retractions, intercostal [re-TRAK-shunz, IN-ter-KOS-tahl] movement of the soft tissue between the ribs inward during inspiration

retractor [ree-TRAK-tor] a surgical instrument used to pull back tissue and structures that would otherwise obscure the view of the surgical field

retro- [ret-row] *prefix*; behind or backward

retrograde [RET-roh-grayd] movement opposite of the normal pattern, moving backward to a less developed or well state

retrograde amnesia [RET-roh-grayd am-NEE-zee-ah] lack of the ability to recall events before the onset of the amnesia

retrograde pyelography [RET-roh-grayd py-eh-LOG-ra-fee] radiological study of the kidneys, ureters, and bladder by injecting a contrast agent

Reye syndrome [RYE SIN-drom] a complex of symptoms following administration of aspirin for fever in children, characterized by liver damage, brain dysfunction, fever, and vomiting

Rh factor [arr-aitch FAK-tor] an antigen found on the surface of red blood cells called Rh-positive; absence of this antigen is indicated by the term Rh-negative

rhabdomyolysis [RAB-doh-my-OL-eye-sis] acute and fulminating destruction of muscle tissue; it is possibly fatal

rhabdomyoma [rab-doh-mih-OH-mah] a nonmalignant tumor of skeletal muscle tissue

rhabdomyosarcoma [rab-doh-MY-oh-sar-KOH-mah] a malignant tumor of striated muscle

rheumatic heart [roo-MAT-ick hart] damage to heart valves as a result of rheumatic fever

rheumatoid arthritis [ROO-mah-toyd arth-RIGH-tis] an acute and chronic autoimmune inflammatory disease of connective tissue that affects joints due to antibodies destroying cartilage at the articular surfaces

rheumatologist [ROO-mah-TAWL-oh-jist] physician who specializes in treating inflammatory and degenerative diseases of connective tissues and joints

rhinencephalon [ryne-en-SEF-ah-lon] anatomical portion of the cerebral cortex associated with the processing of impulses pertaining to smell

rhinitis [RYE-nigh-tis] inflammation of the nasal mucous membrane

rhinophyma [rye-noh-FYE-mah] form of rosacea affecting the nose

rhinoplasty [RHIN-oh-plas-tee] surgical repair of the nose to correct a defect or to change its appearance

rhinorrhagia [RHIN or rhaj ee ah] profuse bleeding from the nose

rhinorrhea [RHIN-or-ree-uh] discharge from the mucous membrane of the nose

rhinovirus [RYE-noh-vy-rus] a large group of viruses that cause upper respiratory infections

rhizotomy [rye-ZAW-toh-mee] incision in a spinal nerve root to relieve intractable pain

rhodopsin [roh-DOP-sin] red pigment of the rods which is bleached by daylight

rhomboideus muscle [rom-BOY-dee-us MUS-sel] muscle that raises and adducts the scapula

rhonchus [RONK-us] harsh, rattling, or whistling sound in lung fields

rhythm [RITH-em] the relative measurement of an impulse or activity in relation to time; regularity of action

rib cage [rib kayg] the bony structure of the thoracic skeleton that is formed by the 12 arched pairs of bone that insert on the sternum

rickets [RIK-etz] childhood disease caused by inadequate vitamin D intake

right atrioventricular valve [rite ay-tree-oh-ven-TRIK-yoo-ler valv] valve between the right ventricle and the right atrium; tricuspid valve

right atrium [rite AYE-tree-um] upper chamber of the heart that receives deoxygenated blood from the entire body except the lungs

right coronary artery [rite KOR-uh-nerr-ee AR-ter-ee] artery supplying blood to the heart tissue

right lung [rite lung] structure of respiration located in the right chest and comprised of the superior and inferior lobes

right ventricle [rite VEN-trih-kul] lower chamber of the heart that receives blood from the right atrium and pumps it out to the lungs by way of the pulmonary artery

rima [RYE-ma] cleft or fissure

Rinne test [RIN-ee test] a method to assess hearing by air conduction by holding a vibrating tuning fork at the base of the mastoid process and the prongs near the ear; normally, patients hear the sound longer by air conduction

ritual [RIH-choo-al] a detailed, prescribed order of actions; may be religious, personal, or part of psychiatric disorders such as obsessive compulsive disorder

rod [RAWD] light-sensitive cell; sensitive to all levels of light but not to color

Romberg's sign [RAWM-bergs sighn] assessing equilibrium by having a patient stand with the feet together and the eyes closed to check for swaying or falling to one side; indicates a loss of balance and inner-ear dysfunction

rongeur [rawn-GHER] a forceps that is used to remove small bone fragments

root [ROOT] a firm structural attachment, often the lowest part of an organ

Rorschach test [ROAR-shahk test] a psychological examination in which a patient is shown cards with abstract shapes and asked to describe what the shape of the inkblot represents; also known as the "inkblot test"

rosacea [roh-ZAY-shee-uh] chronic, noninfectious skin disorder marked by redness on the cheeks, nose, and chin

rosaceiform [roh-ZAY-shee-ih-form] the red mask appearance of cheeks, nose, and skin; typical of rosacea

roseola [ROZ-ee-oh-lah] a rose- or red-colored rash

rotation [roh-TAY-shun] one of the basic movements of a joint; having a quality of turning around an axis

rotator cuff [ROH-tay-tor kuff] collection of muscles that rotate the arm; includes supraspinatus, infraspinatus, teres minor, and subscapularis muscles

rotator cuff tendonitis [ROH-tay-tor kuff ten-don-EYE-tis] inflammation of the tendons of the supraspinatus, infraspinatus, teres minor, or subscapular muscles of the shoulder

round ligament [rownd LIG-ah-ment] residual structures of the umbilical vein found in the liver; a fibromuscular attachment that attaches to the uterus

round window [rownd WIN-doe] a circular, membrane-covered opening in the medial wall of the middle ear leading into the cochlea

Roux-en-Y gastric bypass [roks-en-why GAS-trik BY-pass] surgical treatment of morbid obesity by attaching the jejunum to a surgically reduced stomach pouch and connecting the bypassed duodenum to the pylorus, resulting in decreased gastric capacity and reduced absorption of food

Rovsing's sign [ROV-singz sighn] clinical finding indicating appendicitis whereby pressure in the lower left quadrant of the abdomen produces pain in the lower right quadrant

-rrhage [raj] *suffix*; sudden outpouring of drainage

-rrhagia [raj-ee-ah] *suffix*; sudden outpouring of drainage

-rrhaphy [rah-fee] *suffix*; to suture or sew together

-rrhea [ree-uh] *suffix*; discharge

-rrheic [ree-ik] *suffix*; pertaining to discharge

-rrhexis [rex-is] *suffix*; rupture

rubella [roo-BEL-ah] viral infection; also known as German measles

rubeola [roo-bee-OH-lah] red measles

rubor [ROO-bor] redness which is often associated with infection or inflammation

rugae [ROO-gay] folds and ridges of tissue present in mucous membranes of organs such as the intestine and vagina

rupture [RUP-shur] a tear, break, or protrusion of an organ or body tissue

S

S1 [ess-wun] sound of the heart produced by the closure of the two atrioventricular valves at the start of systole; "lub" sound

S2 [ess-too] sound of the heart produced by the closure of the two semilunar valves at the end of systole; "dub" sound

sacrum [SAY-krum] a group of five fused vertebrae that are not individually numbered, except for the first sacral vertebra (S1); it joins with the hip bones to form the most posterior part of the pelvis

saddle joint [SAD-el JOYNT] articular surface where double motion is due to the concave surface of one joint interacting with the convex surface of another; for example, the carpal and metacarpal of the thumb

saline solution [SAY-leen soh-LOO-shun] an isotonic liquid preparation of salt and distilled water used for infusion or irrigation

saliva [sah-LY-vah] liquid that is secreted by the salivary glands and contains amylase, an enzyme that begins the process of digestion in the oral cavity

salivary amylase [SAL-ih-var-ee AM-ih-lays] an enzyme found in saliva that breaks down starch into simple sugars; produced by the salivary glands

salivary glands [SAL-ih-var-ee glanz] a group of bilaterally located glands (parotid, submandibular, and sublingual) that produce saliva

salpingo-oophorectomy [sal-PING-oh-oof-oh-REK-toh-mee] surgical excision of the fallopian tubes and ovaries

salpingopexy [sal-ping-oh-PEK-see] surgical fixation of a fallopian tube

-salpinx [sal-pinks] *suffix*; pertaining to the fallopian tube

sarcoidosis [sar-koyd-OH-sis] fibrous invasion by granulomatous tissue in the lungs, skin, lymph nodes, spleen, and parotid glands

sarcolemma [sar-koh-LEM-ah] sheath surrounding muscle cell

-sarcoma [sar-koh-ma] *suffix;* a malignant tumor

sarcomeres [SAR-koh-meers] contractile segment of skeletal muscle tissue

sarcoplasm [SAR-koh-plaz-um] intercellular material of the cell, particularly striated muscle cells

sarcosis [sar-KOH-sis] an abnormal formation of skin

sartorius muscle [sar-TOH-ree-us MUS-sel] muscle that flexes the knee and rotates the hip

sartorius quadriceps femoris muscle [sah-TOR-ee-us KWAD-rih-seps FEM-or-is MUS-sel] muscle of the inner thigh that abducts the leg when contracted

scabies [SKAY-beez] mite infection of skin characterized by a pruritic rash due to burrowing habit of the mites

scapula [SKAP-yoo-lah] the large triangular bone of the posterior shoulder; plural is scapulae

scapulodynia [skap-yoo-loh-DIN-ee-ah] painful and inflamed shoulder muscles from injury or overuse

scapulohumeral joint [SKAP-yoo-loh-HEW-mur-ul JOYNT] articular surface between the scapula and humerus; shoulder joint

-schisis [ski-sis] *suffix;* fissure or split

schizophrenia [SKIZ-oh-FREE-nee-ah] a major psychiatric disorder with chronic loss of connection with reality in most or all aspects of life; includes bizarre behavior, disrupted thought processes, hallucinations and delusions of persecution, and alterations in speech

Schwann cell [SHWAN sel] a structure of the peripheral nervous system that forms the myelin sheath and neurilemma of a nerve fiber

sciatica [si-AT-ih-kah] pain that follows the pathway of the sciatic nerve, caused by compression or trauma of the nerve or its roots

scintigram [SIN-teh-gram] nuclear image known as a 3f scintigraphy x-ray

scintigraphy [sin-TIG-rah-fee] injection of a radioactive tracer followed by imagery to detect areas of pathology such as arthritis, fracture, osteomyelitis, or cancerous tumors of the bone

sclera [SKLEER-ah] tough connective tissue that forms a white, continuous layer around the eyeball, functioning to protect the internal structures; plural is sclerae

scleral buckle [SKLEER-ul BUK-kel] a surgically placed band of silicone that acts to permanently tighten the retina

scleredema [skler-eh-DE-mah] edema and redness of the skin that precedes an acute skin infection

scleroderma [skler-oh-DER-mah] a chronic and progressive hardening of skin and connective tissues that produces generalized edema and limitation in movements

scoliosis [SKOH-lee-OH sis] an abnormal lateral curvature of the spine with the original curve and a secondary compensatory curve in the opposite direction

-scope [skohp] *suffix*; instrument for examination

-scopy [skop-ee] *suffix*; examination

scotoma [skoh-TOH-mah] a blind spot in the visual field due to a variety of causes such as glaucoma, diabetic retinopathy, or macular degeneration as nerves are destroyed

scrotal [SKROH-tal] bag; scrotum

scrotum [SKROH-turn] a soft pouch of skin behind the penis containing the testes and part of the spermatic cords

seasonal affective disorder (SAD) [SEE-son-al ah-FEK-tiv dis-OR-der] depression due to hypersecretion of melatonin from the pineal gland in the brain due to decreased intensity and quantity of light during winter months; results in depressed mood, weight gain, and altered sleeping habits

sebaceous cysts [se-BAY-shus SISTS] fluid-filled sebaceous glands

sebaceous glands [se-BAY-shus glanz] structures that secrete sebum to the skin surface

seborrhea [seb-oh-REE-ah] excessive excretion of sebum from the sebaceous glands of the skin

seborrheic dermatitis [seb-oh-REE-ik der-mah-TYE-tis] inflammation of the sebaceous glands of the skin

seborrheic keratosis [seb-oh-REE-ik kair-ah-TOH-sis] benign purple-brown skin tumor(s)

seborrheic warts [seb-or-REE-ik wartz] pigmented skin with a greasy, raised, crusty appearance

second cranial nerve [SEC-ond KRAY-nee-ul nerv] the optic (II) nerve that carries impulses to the brain to deliver input for the sensory function of vision

second-degree burn [SEC-ond-deh-GREE burn] damage to the epidermal and dermal layers

seizure [SEE-zhur] sudden, transient electrical disturbances in the brain resulting from abnormal firing of nerve impulses which may or may not be associated with convulsions

seizure threshold [SEE-zur THRESH-old] level of neurological activity or stimulation that triggers seizure activity

selective serotonin reuptake inhibitors (SSRI) [seh-LEK-tiv ser-oh-TON-in ree-UP-tayk in-HIB-ih-tors] class of antidepressant medications that block the neuronal reuptake of serotonin

semicircular canals [sem-ih-SIR-kyoo-lar kah NALZ] half-circle-shaped structures within the bony labyrinth of the inner ear that are critical to maintaining balance

semicomatose [sem-ee-KOH-mah-tohs] a state near loss of consciousness from which the patient can be aroused

semi-Fowler position [SEH-mee-FOW-ler poe-ZIH-shun] placement of a patient with the head of the bed elevated at least 30 degrees

semilunar bone [sem-ee-LEW-nar bohn] a crescent-shaped bone of the wrist

semilunar valve [sem-ee-LEW-nar valv] half-moon-shaped valve between the heart and the aorta that prevents blood flow from the aorta into the left ventricle during ventricular relaxation

semimembranosus muscle [sem-ee-mem-bruh-NOH-sus MUS-sel] one of three muscles of the posterior thigh that flexes the knee; extends and rotates the hip when contracted

seminal vesicle [SEM-ih-nal VES-ih-kal] structure of the testicle that secretes an alkaline fluid into the ejaculatory duct

seminiferous tubules [SEM-ih-NIF-er-us TOO-byoolz] channels or long tubules located in the testes

semitendinosus muscle [SEM-ee-ten-di-NOH-sus MUS-sel] one of three muscles of the posterior thigh that has a thick tendon attached at the ischium and ends at the medial condyle of the tibia; functions to flex the knee, and extend and rotate the hip

senile plaques [SEE-nyl plaks] clinical finding, associated with Alzheimer's disease, of abnormal amyloid deposits in brain tissue that disrupt brain function

sensorineural hearing loss [SEN-soh-ree-NYOOR-al HEER ing loss] decreased ability to perceive sound due to damage to the hair cells in the cochlea

sensory nerve [SEN-sor-ee nerv] neurological tissue that transmits experiences of sound, light, position, pressure, heat, and cold to the brain

sensory neuron [SEN-sor-ee NYOO-ron] nerves that transmit information back to the central nervous system from the periphery; also known as afferent neuron

sepsis [SEP-sis] an inflammatory response to infection characterized by fever, increased heart and respiratory rates, and decreased blood pressure

septicemia [SEP-tih-SEE-mee-ah] presence of bacterial infection in the blood

septotomy [SEPT-ot-oh-mee] incision into the septum of any dividing structure, especially the nasal septum

septum [SEP-tum] tissue that divides a cavity or space into two parts

sequela [see-KWEL-ah] a condition resulting from a previous disease or disorder; plural is sequelae

seroconversion [SER-oh-kon-VER-shun] process where exposure to a pathogen causes a change from negative to a positive finding of antibodies for that pathogen; often observed with tuberculosis

serotonin [SER-oh-TOH-nin] a neurotransmitter in the central nervous system which stimulates smooth-muscle contraction in the intestinal tract

serous [SEER-us] a watery, serum-like fluid secreted by the serous membrane that is similar to clear liquid serum of the blood

serum gastric test [SEER-um GAS-trik test] laboratory test used to determine level of gastrin in blood serum

serum lipase [SEER-um LIP-ace] test measuring pancreatic enzyme levels of lipase in the blood

sesamoid bone [ses-ah-MOYD bohn] a small ovoid bone embedded in a tendon that lies over a joint and does not articulate with another bone; for example, the patella

sessile polyp [ses-SIL POL-ip] pendulous soft tissue arising from a mucus membrane with a broad base attachment

sexually transmitted disease [SEKS-yoo-al-ee tranz-MIT-tid dis-EEZ] infectious conditions spread by sexual contact, including syphilis, *Chlamydia*, AIDS, gonorrhea, and others

shin splints [SHIN splintz] pain in the anterior tibial region; disorder associated with inflammation and microtears of the tibial periosteum and related extensor muscles due to tremendous muscle stress caused by running on hard surfaces

shingles [SHING-lz] painful raised lesions along nerve roots

short bowel syndrome [short BOW-el SIN-drom] decreased ability to digest and absorb foods due to reduced length of intestine; this may be the result of congenital defects, infection, or extensive necrotizing enterocolitis

sialolith [sigh-AL-oh-lith] stone formed by the body

sialolithiasis [sigh-AL-oh-lith-AYE-sis] a stone formed in the salivary gland which becomes lodged in the duct, blocking the flow of saliva and resulting in painful swelling of the salivary gland, face, or mouth

sialorrhea [sy-ah-loh-REE-ah] excess production of saliva, or increased retention of saliva in the mouth, due to difficulty swallowing

siccant [SIK-ant] agent that removes moisture or promotes dryness of tissue or a body surface

sickle-cell anemia [SIK-kul-SEL ah-NEE-mee-ah] hereditary hemoglobinopathy, with partial or complete replacement of normal hemoglobin with abnormal hemoglobin

sigmoid colon [SIG-moyd KO-lon] an S-shaped section of bowel preceded by the descending colon, terminating at the anus

sigmoidoscope [SIG-moyd-oh-SKOHP] instrument used to visualize the sigmoid colon

silicosis [sil-ih-KOH-sis] pneumoconiosis caused by inhalation of silica dust, often seen in quarry or stone masons who experience occupational exposure

single-photon emission computed tomography [sing-al-FOH-ton ee-MIS-shun kom-PYOO-ted toh-MOG-rah-fee] a nuclear imaging study of organ(s) following the injection of a radioactive tracer

sinoatrial node [sigh-no-AYE-tree-al nohd] a dense network of fibers at the junction of the superior vena cava and the right atrium, where electrical impulses originate

sinus [SY-nus] a cavity or space within a structure

sinus tachycardia [SY-nus tak-ee-KAR-dee-ah] heart rate with normal rhythm but elevated rate above 100 beats per minute

sinusotomy [sy-nus-AW-toh-mee] surgical incision into a sinus

-sis [sis] *suffix*; condition or state

Sjögren syndrome [SHOE-greyn SIN-drom] autoimmune disease marked by dry skin, dry nasal membranes, and multiple areas of arthritis

skeletal traction [SKEL-eh-tal TRAK-shun] use of pins, wires, or tongs inserted into the bone during surgery to align the bone fragments

skin traction [skin TRAK-shun] use of elastic wraps, straps, halters, or skin adhesives connected to a pulley and weights, to align a body part following surgery or a fracture

sleep apnea [sleep AP-nee-uh] cessation of breathing during sleep that causes awakening and is characterized by daytime sleepiness

slit-lamp examination [SLIT-lamp ex-am-in-AY-shun] diagnostic procedure to detect abnormalities of the cornea, anterior chamber, iris, or lens using a low-power microscope (biomicroscope) for magnification with a high-intensity light

socket [SOH-kit] a hollow joint or acetabulum

soleus muscle [SOH-lee-us MUS-sel] muscle of the foot that causes plantar flexion when contracted

soma [SOH-muh] all cells in the body except bacteria

somatization [so-mah-ti-ZAY-shun] process of expressing emotional distress by physical complaints

somatostatin [SOH-mah-to-STAT-in] a peptide responsible for the regulation and inhibition of hormones by various neuroendocrine cells in the brain and gastrointestinal tract

-some [sohm] *suffix*; body

somnolent [SOM-no-lent] prolonged drowsiness, sedation, or sleepiness, often the result of disease or medications

-spasm [spa-zim] *suffix*; sudden, involuntary contraction

spastic athetosis [SPAZ-tik ath-eh-TOH-sis] constant involuntary writhing motions that are most often due to an extrapyramidal lesion

spastic paralysis [spaz-TIK pa-RAL-ih-sis] stiff and awkward muscle control caused by a central nervous system disorder

specific gravity [spe-SIF-ik GRAV-ih-tee] measure of the density of the urine compared to that of water

spermatic [sper-MAT-ik] pertaining to spermatozoon

spermatogenesis [SPER-mah-toh-JEN-eh-sis] the process of forming mature spermatozoa

spermatozoa [SPER-mah-tah-ZOH-ah] a mature sperm cell

sphincter [SFINGK-ter] a muscle that encircles a duct or tube in such a manner that constriction closes the orifice or lumen

sphincter of Oddi [SFINK-ter uv OD-ee] a circular muscle in the common bile duct that opens to permit passage of bile and pancreatic secretions into the duodenum

sphygmomanometer [sfing-moh-man-OM-et-ur] instrument used to measure blood pressure in millimeters of mercury; abbreviated mm Hg

sphygmus [SFIG-mus] pulse or pulsating quality

spica hip cast [SPY-kah hip kast] a rigid cast of the lower torso extending to one or both of the legs; used for femoral fractures

spina bifida [SPYE-nah BIF-ih-duh] a congenital defect resulting in incomplete closure of the vertebral column, usually in the lumbosacral region

spina bifida cystica [SPYE-nah BIF-ih-duh SIS-ti-kuh] the most severe type of spina bifida, characterized by increased intracranial pressure, meningocele, hydrocephalus, paraplegia, and the inability to control urinary bladder or rectum

spina bifida occulta [SPYE-nah BIF-ih-duh oh-KULT-ah] incomplete fusion of the vertebral posterior arch without protrusion as the lesion is covered by skin and generally evident only on x-ray evaluation

spinal [SPY-nal] pertaining to the backbone or vertebrae

spinal cord [SPY-nal kord] major nervous tissue originating at the base of the skull and terminating at the area between the first and third lumbar vertebra

spinal nerves [SPY-nal nervs] the 31 paired nerves originating from the spinal cord and containing afferent and efferent fibers to send and receive nervous impulses

spine [SPYN] vertical column of bones composed of 24 individual vertebrae plus the sacrum and coccyx

spiral fracture [SPY-ral FRAK-shur] this fracture occurs when a bone is broken because of a twisting force

spleen [SPLEEN] a nonvital, highly vascular organ involved with lymphocyte production; located in the left hypochondriac region

splenectomy [spleen-NEK-toh-mee] surgical removal of the spleen when it has ruptured due to trauma

splenic vein [SPLEN-ik vayn] vascular structure that carries deoxygenated blood away from the spleen to the portal vein

splenius capitis muscle [SPLEE-nee-us KAP-ih-tis MUS-sel] a muscle of the dorsal surface of the head that, when contracted, pulls the head into an upright position

splenocele [SPLEE-noh-seel] herniation of the spleen

splenomegaly [SPLEN-oh-MEG-ah-lee] enlargement of the spleen, detectable with palpation of the abdomen; possible causes are mononucleosis, Hodgkin's disease, hemolytic anemia, polycythemia vera, and leukemia

splenorrhaphy [splee-NOR-ah-fee] profuse bleeding from the spleen due to laceration or rupture

spondylolisthesis [SPAWN-dih-LOH-lis-THEE-sis] degenerative condition of the spine in which one vertebra moves anteriorly due to degeneration of the intervertebral disc; often due to traumatic injury or compression fracture of the vertebra from osteoporosis

spontaneous fracture [spawn-TAY-nee-us FRAK-shur] breakage of a bone resulting from an underlying disease such as osteoporosis

sprain [SPRAYN] overstretching or tearing of a ligament; treated by rest, immobilization, or surgery to repair the ligament

sputum [SPEW-tum] fluid or semifluid material discharged from the mouth, air passages, and throat

squamous cell carcinoma [SKWAY-mus sell kahr-si-NOH-muh] cancer that develops in the epidermis

ST interval [ess-tee IN-ter-val] segment of an electrocardiogram tracing that indicates time between ventricular contractions

-stalsis [stal-sis] *suffix*; contraction

staphylococcus [STAF-ih-loh-KOK-kus] a class of bacterium that has a characteristic clumping quality similar to a cluster of grapes; causes pyrogenic infections

Starling's law of the heart [STAR-lingz law uv the HART] the force of heart contraction is determined by the length of cardiac heart muscle fibers, and therefore, the further they stretch during diastole, the greater the force of the heartbeat

-stasis [stay-sis] *suffix*; standstill, or unmoving

stasis dermatitis [STAY-sis der-mah-TY-tis] inflammation of and increased pigmentation and thickening of the skin of the lower extremities due to decreased venous return

statins [STA-tinz] a pharmacological class of agents that reduce low-density lipids (LDL)

status asthmaticus [STA-tus az-MAT-ih-kus] a prolonged, extremely severe, life-threatening asthma attack

steatoma [stee-ah-TOH-mah] lipoma, fatty tumor

steatorrhea [stee-AT-oh-REE-uh] greasy, frothy, foul-smelling stools that contain undigested fats

-stenosis [sten-oh-sis] *suffix*; narrowed or constricted

stereocilia [ster-ee-oh-SIL-ee-ah] hair cells located in the inner ear; the hairs are involved with balance and equilibrium

stereognosis [ster-ee-og-NOH-sis] mental ability to perceive the form and nature of objects by touch; tested as part of neurological assessment

stereoscopic vision [ster-ee-oh-SKOP-ik VIH-zhun] three-dimensional vision with depth perception

sternal [STER-nal] pertaining to the breastbone

sternal retraction [STER-nal re-TRAK-shun] inward movement of the breastbone associated with respiratory distress syndrome

sternocleidomastoid muscle [STER-noh-klye-doh-MAS-toyd MUS-sel] muscle that flexes the neck in a forward motion

sternohyoid muscle [ster-noh-HIGH-oyd MUS-sel] a muscle that extends from the medial aspect of the clavicle and sternum to the hyoid bone of the neck and depresses the hyoid bone and larynx when contracted

sternum [STER-num] long, narrow, flat bone of the medial chest; breastbone

Stevens-Johnson syndrome [STEE-venz-JON-son SIN-drom] a systemic skin disorder with fever and blistering lesions of the skin and of all mucous membranes, including the mouth and conjunctivae, resulting in dehydration, infection, sepsis, and possibly death

stimulation [STIM-yoo-LAY-shun] the irritating or arousing of muscles, nerves, or other sensory organs

stockinet [stok-in-ET] a tubular elastic mesh device that holds dressings in place on the trunk, head, and extremities

stoma [STOH-mah] an artificially created opening on the surface of the body, such as a colostomy or tracheostomy

stomach [STUM-ak] a muscular structure that is situated between the esophagus and duodenum, and secretes hydrochloric acid and other digestive juices

stomatitis [STO-mah-TY-tis] inflammation of the oral mucosa which can be caused by poorly fitting dentures that rub the gums

-stomy [stohm-ee] *suffix;* creation of an artificial opening

strabismus [strah-BIZ-mus] disorder of the eye alignment where one eye deviates from the point of focus

strangulated hernia [STRANG-yoo-lay-ted HUR-nee-ah] abnormal protrusion of the intestine through the abdominal wall, obstructing blood flow and fecal movement

stratum [STRAY-tum] a thin layer of tissue having uniform thickness

strawberry hemangioma [STRAW-ber-ee he-man-jee-OH-muh] type of birthmark characterized by raised vascular nevus, commonly observed on the face or neck

stress fracture [STRESS FRAK-shur] fine-line disruption of bone integrity due to repetitive microtrauma

stressor [STRES-or] negative and positive life events

stria [STRY-uh] narrow marking band on skin; stretch marks

striated muscle [STRY-aye-ted MUS-sel] skeletal and cardiac muscles showing bands of color when examined under the microscope

stricture [STRIK-chur] constriction or narrowing of a lumen, duct, or organ such as the urethra, ureter, or esophagus

stridor, respiratory [STRY-dor, RES-pih-ra-tor-ee] an abnormally high-pitched sound during inspiration due to the constriction or narrowing of the larynx or trachea

strumectomy [stru-MEK-toh-mee] surgical excision of a portion or all of a tumor on the thyroid gland

Stryker frame [STRY-ker fraym] a structure that holds the patient on a bed; it can be rotated into different positions while keeping the patient's body from moving

sub- [sub] *prefix*; under or below

subarachnoid space [sub-ah-RAK-ah-noyd spays] the cerebrospinal fluid-filled area between the pia mater and the arachnoid surfaces of the brain

subclavian artery [sub-KLAY-vee-an AR-ter-ee] blood vessel that supplies oxygenated blood to the brain and face; palpable pulsation is called the subclavian pulse

subclavian vein [sub-KLAY-vee-an vayn] a large blood vessel that drains in the arm, joining with the internal jugular vein

subclinical [sub-KLIN-ih-kal] having mild or subtle indications of a disorder

subcutaneous [sub-kew-TAY-nee-us] connective tissue skin layer; hypodermis

subdural [sub-DUR-ahl] space between the dura mater and arachnoid matter of the brain

sublingual (SL) [sub-LIN-gwal] pertaining to the oral mucosal surface immediately under the tongue; often used as a delivery modality for medications in which the medication is allowed to dissolve under the tongue

sublingual glands [sub-LIN-gwal glandz] lymph nodules that drain the region of the throat and tonsils

subluxation [sub-luk-SAY-shun] incomplete dislocation where the articular surfaces are out of normal alignment but still in contact with each other

submandibular [sub-man-DIB-yoo-lar] pertaining to the area under the lower jaw

submandibular nodes [sub-man-DIB-yoo-lar nohdz] lymphatic tissue immediately beneath the lower jaw

submandibularitis [sub-man-DIB-yoo-lar-EYE-tis] inflammation of the lymph nodes below the lower jaw due to bacterial infection; commonly associated with mumps

submental lymph nodes [sub-MEN-tal LYMF nohdz] lymph nodes located under the chin that drain and circulate lymph from the head and throat region

subscapularis muscle [sub-SKAP-yoo-lahr-is MUS-sel] muscle that medially rotates the shoulder

subtalar joint [sub-TAY-lar joynt] articular surface between the talus and calcaneus bones of the foot

subtendinous iliac bursa [sub-TEN-dih-nus ILL-ee-ak BUR-sah] the sheath covering at the point of attachment for the iliopsoas muscle to the lesser trochanter of the femoral head

sucrase [SOO-krays] enzyme secreted by the small intestine to break sucrose into glucose

sudoresis [sue-doh-REE-sis] profuse sweating or perspiration

sudoriferous glands [sue-doh-RIF-er-us glandz] structures that produce sweat

suffocative goiter [SUF-oh-kay-tiv GOY-ter] enlargement of the thyroid gland that presses on the upper airway, producing respiratory stridor

suggillation [sug-ji-LAY-shun] bleeding under the skin; bruising

suicidal ideation [soo-ih-SY-dal EYE-dee-aye-shun] to entertain thoughts or make plans to end one's own life

sundowning [SUN-dow-ning] increased level of confusion, restlessness, and confusion in the late afternoon and evening hours in patients with dementia

super- [sue-per] *prefix*; above, high, or excessive

superficial [SUE-per-FISH-al] near the surface; shallow, not deep or penetrating

superior [soo-PEER-ee-or] situated above another structure; of higher quality

superior hepatic vein [soo-PEER-ee-or he-PAH-tik vayn] major blood vessel that moves blood away from the liver and intestinal tract

superior oblique muscle [soo-PEER-ee-or ob-LEEK MUS-sel] muscle that turns the eye upward and toward the midline of the visual field

superior rectus muscle [soo-PEER-ee-or REK-tus MUS-sel] muscle that turns the eye upward

superior vena cava [soo-PEER-ee-or VEE-na KAY-vah] large vessel that returns blood from the head, neck, and upper limbs, terminating at the right atrium

supinator muscle [SOO-pi-nay-tur MUS-sel] muscle that turns the forearm in a palm down position

supine [SOO-pyne] positioning of a patient lying on the back with the palms facing up

suppository [suh-PAWS-ih-tor-ee] a formed, bullet-shaped capsule that contains a drug for administration of medication by melting in the rectum where it is absorbed

supra- [sue-prah] *prefix*; above or excessive

supra spinatus muscle [SOO-prah spye-NAY-tus MUS-sel] muscle that abducts the shoulder

suprapubic catheter [sue-prah-PEW-bik KATH-eh-ter] insertion of a catheter into the bladder above the symphysis pubis bone using a surgical incision

suprapubic prostatectomy [soo-prah-PYOO-bik praws-tah-TEK-toh-mee] excision of the prostate gland by a superior approach above the symphysis pubis to avoid nerves to the penis

suprarenal glands [sue-pra-REE-nal glanz] an excretory structure that produces epinephrine, norepinephrine, and cortisone; also regulates carbohydrate metabolism, salt, and water balance

supraventricular tachycardia [SOO-prah-ven-TRIK-yoo-lar TAK-ee-KAR-dee-uh] common pathologic tachycardia characterized by abrupt onset of a rapid, regular heart rate, often too fast to count

surfactant [sur-FAK-tant] agent that lowers the surface tension of a liquid, such as mucous in the upper airway

suspensory ligaments [suh-SPENS-or-ee LIG-ah-mentz] fibrous tissue that serves the purpose of holding structures, such as the ovary and uterus, in anatomical position

Swan-Ganz catheter [swan-ganz KATH-eh-ter] a flexible catheter inserted into the pulmonary artery of patients in shock; used for hemodynamic monitoring

sym- [sim] *prefix*; with or together

sympathetic ganglion [sym-pah-THEH-tik GANG-lee-on] a collection of nerve cells that are attached to efferent fibers that originate from visceral motor neurons in the thoracic and upper lumbar spine

symphysis pubis [SIM-fi-sis PEW-bis] the fibrocartilaginous union of the pubic bones

symptom [SIMP-tom] a change in health experienced by a patient

symptomology [SIMP-tom-AWL-oh-jee] clinical representation of signs and symptoms associated with a disease

syn- [sin] *prefix*; with or together

synapse [SIN-aps] communicating region between neurons

synaptic cleft [syn-AP-tik kleft] a small, fluid-filled space between two neurons where neurotransmitters are released

synaptic terminal [syn-AP-tik TER-mih-nal] the end portion of an axon that receives the nerve impulse

synaptic vesicle [syn-AP-tik VES-ih-kl] a small, saclike structure at the end of the synapse that contains neurotransmitters

synchia [syn-KEE-ah] adhesion of tissues, particularly the iris, lens, and cornea

synchondrosis [sin-kon-DROH-sis] joint in which the surfaces are connected by a cartilage plate

syncope [SING-koh-pee] loss of consciousness due to inadequate oxygen to the brain

syndactyly [sin-DAK-tih-lee] congenital condition in which soft tissues of fingers or toes are joined

syndesmosis [syn-dez-MOH-sis] articulation in which the bones are held together by fibrous connective tissue

syndesmotomy [syn-des-MOT-oh-mee] surgical incision of ligaments

syndrome [SIN-drom] signs and symptoms of a particular disease

synechotomy [syn-ek-OT-oh-mee] surgical incision of an adhesion

synechtenterotomy [syn-EK-ten-ter-OT-oh-mee] surgical excision of adhesions of the intestine

syphilis [SIF-ih-lis] multiphase, sexually transmitted disease caused by infection with the organism *Treponema pallidum*

syrigmus [sir-IG-mus] subjective report of ringing or hissing sounds in the ears

systematic desensitization [sis-teh-MAT-ik dee-SEN-sih-tih-ZAY-shun] a technique in which a patient imagines multiple scenarios of progressively greater anxiety while utilizing relaxation techniques until they no longer cause anxiety; used as an adjunct to pharmacological therapies in treating severe anxiety

systemic [SIS-tem-ik] relating to the whole body

systemic lupus erythematosus (SLE) [sis-TEM-ik LOU-pus eh-rith-mah-TOH-sis] a chronic autoimmune inflammatory disease with characteristic facial "butterfly rash," involving hematologic, cardiac, pulmonary, and renal systems

systole [SIS-toh-lee] contraction of the heart muscle

systolic blood pressure [sis-TOL-ik BLUD presh-ur] arterial blood pressure during ventricular contraction

T

T wave [TEE wayv] section of the electrocardiogram (ECG) showing ventricular repolarization

tachy- [tak-ee] *prefix*; swift or rapid

tachycardia [tak-ee-KAHR-dee-ah] rapid heart rate in excess of 100 beats per minute

tachyphylaxis [tak-ee-fil-AX-is] rapid loss of a therapeutic response to a pharmacological agent

tachypnea [tak-ip-NEE-uh] rapid respiratory rate

tactile stimulation [TAK-tile stim-yoo-LAY-shun] invoking a neurological response by touching

talipes equinovarus [TAY-lih-peez ee-KWY-noh-VAR-us] congenital deformity of one or both feet in which the foot is pulled downward and laterally; the heel never rests on the floor, causing the patient to walk on the toes; most common type of clubfoot

talus [TAY-lus] the first tarsal bone and the largest of the bones of the ankle, which articulates with the tibia and fibula

tardive dyskinesia [TAR-dive DIS-kih-NEE-zee-ah] a complication of treatment with antipsychotic medications that produces abnormal, involuntary, repetitive movements of the face (grimacing, lip smacking, eye blinking, tongue movements) and can also include movements of the arms and legs

Tarlov cysts [TAHR-lov sistz] perineural cysts located in the proximal radicles of the lower spinal cord which produce symptoms of nerve pain

tarsal [TAR-sol] pertaining to the seven individual bones that make up the ankle

T-cells [TEE-sells] thymus-derived lymphocytes that recognize and kill cancerous cells and cells infected with viruses or identified as foreign tissue

temporal artery [tem-POR-al AR-ter-ee] blood vessel that brings oxygenated blood to the brain

temporal bone [tem-POR-al bohn] segment of the cranium located on the sides of the head, anterior to the ears

temporal foramen [TEM-poh-ral FOR-aye-men] a small opening in the cranium for the ear canal

temporal lobe [tem-POR-al lohb] lateral segments of the cerebrum under the temporal bone

temporalis muscle [tem-poh-RAL-is MUS-sel] smooth muscle of the lateral surface of the face

temporomandibular joint syndrome [TEM-poh-roh-man DIB-yoo-lar JOYNT SIN-drom] dysfunction of the temporomandibular joint with clicking, pain, muscle spasm, and difficulty opening the jaw; caused by chewing on only one side of the mouth, clenching or grinding the teeth during sleep, or misalignment of the teeth

tendolysis [ten-DOL-eye-is] releasing a tendon from adhesions

tendons [TEN-dunz] fibrous bands or cords that attach muscle to bone or muscle to other body parts

tendoplasty [TEN-do-plas-tee] surgical repair of a tendon to restore functionality

tenotomy [teh-NOT-oh-mee] surgical resection of a tendon

tensor fasciae latae muscle [TEN-sor FASH-ee-aye LAY-tah MUS-sel] muscle of the hip that extends the hip when contracted

teratogenic [ter-ah-toh-JEN-ik] affecting the development of a fetus, as in transmitting or causing malformation

teres major muscle [TEER-eez MAY-jor MUS-sel] muscle that extends and medially rotates shoulder

teres minor muscle [TEER-eez MY-nohr MUS-sel] muscle that rotates the arm laterally

terminal [TER-mih-nal] pertaining to the end boundary, especially a disease from which a patient cannot recover or that is likely to cause death

testicle [TES-tih-kul] male gonad which functions to produce sperm and testosterone; singular form of testes

testosterone [tes-TAWS-ter-rohn] sex hormone responsible for masculine characteristics: maturation of sexual organs, spermatogenesis, sex drive, erectile capabilities, facial hair, and pronounced musculature

tetanus [TET-ah-nus] infection with the bacillus *Clostridium tetani* in deep puncture wounds; characterized by gross muscular rigidity, severe muscle spasms, respiratory failure, and death

tetany [TET-ah-nee] painful intermittent muscle spasms frequently associated with calcium imbalance

tetra- [tet-rah] *prefix*; four

tetraiodothyronine [tet-rah-eye-oh-doh-THIGH-roh-nine] thyroid hormone

tetralogy of Fallot [te-TRAL-oh-jee uv fahl-OH] four congenital heart defects appearing together

tetranopsia [tet-rah-NOP-see-ah] loss of one-fourth of the visual field

tetraparesis [tet-rah-PAR-ee-sis] muscular weakness in all four extremities

thalamus [THAL-ah-mus] gray matter on either side of the third ventricle of the brain that acts as a relay station for impulses from the sensory nerves and sends them to specific cortical areas of the brain

thallium [THAL-ee-um] assessment of coronary artery disease by use of a radioactive isotope of thallium administered by an intravenous drip, followed by a physical stress test; the isotope collects in areas of decreased circulation and can be visualized on the scanner

thanatophobia [THAN-ah-toh-FOH-bee-ah] fear of death

therapy vest [THER-ah-pee vest] a vestlike garment that vibrates, shaking the chest wall in efforts to break up mucus from lung fields for expectoration or suctioning

thermoreceptor [ther-moh-ree-SEP-tor] sensory sites that are stimulated by the rise in temperature

thermoregulation [THER-moh-reg-yoo-LAY-shun] efforts by the hypothalamus to maintain body temperature by heat production and heat loss

theta waves [THAY-tah wayvz] brain waves seen on electroencephalography; most often found in children, but may occur in adults under emotional stress

thimerosal [thigh-MER-oh-sal] a mercury compound used to preserve pharmacological agents and vaccines

third-degree burn [third-deh-GREE burn] destruction of the full thickness of the skin and underlying structures due to chemical or thermal exposure

thoracentesis [THOR-ah-sen-TEE-sis] removal of fluid from the thoracic cavity, usually due to cancer or pneumonia

thoracic [thoh-RAS-ik] pertaining to the chest

thoracic lymph duct [thoh-RAS-ik LIMF dukt] the common trunk of all lymphatic vessels in the body except those from the right neck and head area

thoracic outlet compression syndrome [thoh-RAS-ik OUT-let kom-PRESH-un SIN-drom] compression of nerves and/or blood vessels of the neck due to entrapment between the pectoralis minor and adjacent muscles, resulting in decreased sensation and blood supply to the upper extremities

thoracic spine [thoh-RAS-ik SPYN] the region of the 12 bony segments of the spinal column of the upper back, designated T1 to T12

thoracic vertebrae [thoh-RAS-ik VER-teh-bray] the 12 discs of the spinal column that connect the ribs, forming the posterior wall of the thorax

thoracocentesis [thor-ah-koh-sen-TEE-sis] removal of fluid from the chest cavity using a surgical puncture, usually a large-bore needle

thoracometer [tho-rah-KOM-eh-ter] medical device used to measure the expansion of the chest during inspiration

thoracoplasty [THOR-ah-koh-plas-tee] surgical removal of portions of the ribs to collapse diseased portions of the lung in efforts to treat pulmonary tuberculosis and empyema

thoracotomy [thor-ah-KOT-oh-mee] surgical incision of the chest wall, usually performed laterally between the ribs

thorax [THOR-aks] portion of the body below the base of the neck and above the diaphragm; further divided into the anterior, posterior, and axillary surfaces

thromboangiitis obliterans [throm-boh-an-jee-EYE-tis uh-BLIT-ur-anz] inflammation and decreased blood flow in the peripheral arteries and veins of the extremities

caused by long-term tobacco use; also known as
Buerger disease

thrombocytopenia [THRAWM-boh-sy-toh-PEE-nee-ah]
deficiency of thrombocytes due to action or chemicals
or drugs that damage stem cells in the bone marrow;
also occurs when leukemia cells take over and crowd
the stem cells that produce thrombocytes

thrombocytosis [throm-boh-sy-TOH-sis] mildly increased
number of platelets in circulation

thrombolytic [throm-boh-LIT-ik] dissolution of blood clots
by breaking down the fibrin strands

thrombophlebitis [throm-boh-fleb-EYE-tis] vein
inflammation and thrombus (clot) formation

thrombosis [throm-BOH-sis] formation or presence of a clot
in a blood vessel

thymectomy [thigh-MEK-toh-mee] surgical removal of the
thymus due to a tumor or myasthenia gravis

-thymia [thigh-mee-uh] *suffix*; state of mind

thymoma [thigh-MOH-mah] a tumor of the thymus which
is usually benign

thymosins [THIGH-moh-sins] an endocrine gland that
produces lymphocytes and regulates the immune
system; located posterior to the sternum between
the lungs

thymus [THIGH-mus] a lymph organ located in the
anterosuperior mediastinum

thyroid [THIGH-roid] the gland that secretes thyroid
hormones

thyroid cancer [THIGH-royd KAN-ser] malignant neoplasm
of the thyroid gland; there are four types: papillary,
follicular, medullary, and undifferentiated; treatment
has a very high success rate

thyroid cartilage [THIGH-royd KAR-tih-laj] V-shaped
structure surrounding the larynx that forms a

subcutaneous projection; commonly referred to as the "Adam's apple"

thyroid scan [THIGH-royd skan] diagnostic nuclear scan in which a radioactive substance is injected and uptake by the thyroid gland is measured using a gamma camera

thyroid stimulating hormone (TSH) [THIGH-royd STIM-yoo-lay-ting HOR-mohn] substance secreted by the pituitary gland that triggers the thyroid gland to produce thyroxine and triiodothyronine

thyroidectomy [thigh-royd-EK-toh-mee] partial or complete surgical removal of the thyroid gland

thyrotoxic [THIGH-roh-TOK-sik] crisis exacerbation of the symptoms of hyperthyroidism; thyroid storm

thyrotoxicosis [thigh-roh-tok-si-KOH-sis] condition of excessive thyroid hormone

thyroxine (T_4) [THIGH-roks-in] one of the hormones secreted by the thyroid gland responsible for metabolic rate and processing of all types of food and protein synthesis in bodily tissues

tibia [TIB-ee-ah] small bone of the anterior surface of the lower leg

tibialis anterior muscle [tib-ee-AH-lis an-TEER-ee-or MUS-sel] muscle of the anterior lower leg that flexes the foot and ankle when contracted

tibialis muscle [tib-ee-AL-is MUS-sel] acts to produce anterior inversion of the foot

tibiofemoral joint [tib-ee-oh-FEM-uh-rul JOYNT] the articular surface of the tibia and femur; knee joint

-tic [tik] *suffix*; pertaining to

tidal volume (TV) [TYE-dal VOL-yoom] volume of air moved in or out of the lungs during normal breathing

tinea [TIN-ee-uh] lesions of dermatophytoses which may present in the feet (pedi), nails (unguium), groin area (cruris), or any superficial skin surface (versicolor)

Tinel's test [tih-NELZ test] assessment for carpal tunnel syndrome where the patient's arms are tapped with a reflex hammer; positive report of "pins and needles" sensation is diagnostic for carpal tunnel syndrome

tinnitus [tin-EYE-tus] ringing sensation in the ear

-tion [shun] *suffix*; condition or state

tissue plasminogen activator [TISH-yoo plaz-MIN-oh-jen AK-tih-vay-tor] an enzymatic substance that acts to dissolve blood clots; used therapeutically following myocardial infarction to restore blood supply to heart muscle

titer [TY-ter] a standardized measurement of the concentration of a substance in a solution; often used to measure the presence of immune response to vaccinations

-tocia [toh-see-ah] *suffix*; labor; to give birth

tocolysis [toh-koh-LYE-sis] inhibition or prevention of uterine contractions in efforts to delay delivery of a fetus

tolerance [TAWL-er-ans] progressive decrease in therapeutic effect of a drug or therapy

-tome [tohm] *suffix*; instrument used for a particular purpose

tomography [toh-MOG-rah-fee] procedure of making a radiographic image of a selected physical plane for diagnostic purposes

-tomy [toh-mee] *suffix*; incision or cut

tongue [TUNG] muscular organ of the mouth involved with taste and management of oral secretions

tonic [TAWN-ik] continuous muscular contraction; often used to describe seizure activity

tonic-clonic movements [TAWN-ik-KLAWN-ik MOOV-mentz] stiffening and jerking of all major motor muscle groups; previously known as grand-mal seizure

tonometry [toh-NAWM-eh-tree] diagnostic procedure to detect increased intraocular pressure indicative of glaucoma

torsade de pointes [tor-SAHD deh point] a rapid and unstable type of ventricular tachy cardia characterized by shifts in the QRS complex in a manner that appears to shift or twist

tonsillectomy [ton-sih-LEK-toh-mee] surgical excision of the tonsils

tonsillitis [TAWN-sih-LY-tis] acute or chronic bacterial infection of the palatine tonsils and pharynx producing difficulty swallowing, edema and hypertrophy of tonsillar crypts, and blockage of the eustachian tubes

tonsils [TAWN-silz] lymphatic tissue located at the back of the throat that detect and respond to infection of the throat

torpid [TOR-pid] sluggish movements and/or slowed reactions due to neurological pathology such as drug side effects, anoxia, or brain trauma; also, sluggish or delayed responses associated with Parkinson's disease

Tourette's syndrome [TOOR-etz SIN-drom] frequent, spontaneous, involuntary body-movement tics (eye blinking, throat clearing, arm thrusting) and vocal tics (grunts, barks), or comments that are socially inappropriate, vulgar, or obscene

torticollis [tor-tih-KOL-is] stiff, spasmodic neck typically producing lateral flexion of the muscles of the cervical spine

tortuous [TOR-choo-us] twisted, sinuous, wavy; as seen in varicose veins

total anomalous pulmonary venous return [TOH-tal ah-NOM-ah-lus PUHL-moh-nair-ee VEE-nus ree-TURN] a congenital heart defect in which the pulmonary veins empty into the right atrium or veins leading to the right atrium

total lung capacity (TLC) [TOE-tal lung ka-PAS-ih-tee] volume of air that the lungs can hold, defined as the vital capacity combined with the residual volume; average value = 6,000 cc

toxigenicity [toks-ih-jen-IS-ih-tee] relative potency of a poison-producing organism

trabecular meshwork [trah-BEK-yoo-lar MESH-wurk] area of interlacing fibers in which the aqueous humor is filtered; located in the region where the edges of the iris and the cornea meet

trabeculoplasty [trah-BEK-yoo-loh-PLAS-tee] surgical procedure used to treat glaucoma, where an argon laser is used to create small holes in half of the trabecular meshwork to increase the flow of aqueous humor

trachea [TRAY-kee-ah] a round cartilaginous structure of the upper airway that extends from the larynx to the bronchiole tubes

trachealis muscle [tray-kee-AH-lis MUS-sel] a muscle of the throat that decreases the lumen of the tracheal rings when contracted

trachelodynia [tray-keh-loh-DIN-ee-uh] pain in the neck

trachelokyphosis [tray-keh-low-ky-FOH-sis] abnormal or excessive anterior curvature of the cervical neck

tracheobronchial suction [TRAY-kee-oh-BRON-kee-al SUK-shun] use of a cannula to remove mucus, pus, or aspirated material from the trachea and upper bronchus to improve air exchange

tracheobronchial tree [TRAY-ke-oh-BRONK-ee-al tree] the inverted treelike structure of the trachea, main stem bronchi, and bronchioles; also known as bronchial tree

tracheomalacia [TRAY-kee-oh-ma-LAY-sha] degeneration of elastic and connective tissues in the trachea

tracheostenosis [TRAY-kee-oh-sten-OH-sis] narrowing of the lumen of the trachea

tracheostomy [TRAY-kee-AWS-toh-mee] an incision into the trachea creating a permanent opening to allow for a patent or open airway

traction [TRAK-shun] the process of putting a limb, bone, or group of muscles under tension by means of weights and pulleys to align or immobilize the part to reduce muscle spasm or to relieve pressure

tragus [TRAY-gus] the small frontal portion of ear cartilage near the auditory canal

tranquilizer [TRAN-kwih-LYZ-er] a major class of drugs used to relieve anxiety and tension, ranging from benzodiazepines to neuroleptics

trans- [trahns] *prefix*; across or through

transcatheter closure [tranz-KATH-eh-ter KLOH-zur] repair of a septal defect using a septal occluder or Rashkind device during cardiac catheterization

transcutaneous electrical nerve stimulation (TENS) [TRANS-kyoo-TAY-nee-us ee-LEK-trik-al nerv stim-yoo-LAY-shun] application of mild electrical current to the skin over a painful region, providing pain relief by interfering with transmission of pain signals

transdermal [trans-DERM-al] administration or absorption of a drug through intact skin

transesophageal echocardiography [TRAS-eh-sof-uh-GEE-al ek-oh-kar-dee-OG-rah-fee] examination of the heart using an endoscope and sonographic transducer inserted in the esophagus directly behind the heart

transferrin [trans-FAIR-in] blood chemistry test to determine the total iron-binding capacity of the blood

transfusion [trans-FYOO-zhun] injection of solutions, blood, and/or chemotherapeutic agents into a vein for therapeutic purposes

transient ischemic attack [tran-SEE-ent is-KEE-mik ah-TAK] temporary interference with blood supply to the brain by small clots, causing no permanent brain damage

transmyocardial revascularization [tranz-my-oh-KAR-dy-al ree-VASK-u-lar-eye-zay-shun] abbreviated TMR, use of a laser to open small channels in the heart muscle to restore blood flow in patients with angina associated with advanced coronary artery disease. This procedure is used when other surgical interventions are not viable.

transplantation [TRANZS-plan-TAY-shun] implantation of a living body part, organ, or tissue graft from a donor

transposition of the great arteries (TGA) [tranz-poh-SIZH-shun uv the grayt AR-ter-eez] condition where the pulmonary artery is the outflow for left ventricle, and the aorta is the outflow for right ventricle; life-threatening at birth, and survival initially depends on open ducts of arteriosus and foramen ovale; this condition occurs in about 5 percent of children with congenital heart disease

transsexualism [tranz-SEK-shoo-ah-lizm] belief of an individual that he or she has been assigned (by anatomy, parents, or society) the wrong gender identity, and needs to change his or her outward appearance to the opposite sex in order to match what is already felt in the mind

transurethral resection [TRANS-yoo-REE-thral ree-SEK-shun] the surgical removal of a structure performed through the urethra

transverse [trans-VERS] a horizontal plane that divides the body into two sections: upper and lower

transverse fracture [trans-VERS FRAK-shur] a bone break that is perpendicular to the bone's long axis

transversus abdominis muscle [trans-VUR-sus ab-DOM-ih-nis MUS-sel] muscle that compresses the abdomen and aids in posture

trapezium [tra-PEE-zee-um] a four-sided bone of the wrist that articulates with the base of the thumb

trapezius muscle [trah-PEE-zee-us MUS-sel] a flat, triangular muscle of the posterior shoulder and neck that shrugs the shoulder when flexed

tremor [TREM-or] involuntary shaking of a body part due to pathological states such as Parkinson's disease or side effects of medications; some subtypes include intention, coarse, fine, and resting, often detected in the hands and upper body

Trendelenburg position [tren-DEL-en-berg po-SISH-un] placement of a patient lying flat in bed with the head lowered and the feet elevated to enhance blood flow to the brain and vital organs

tri- [try] *prefix*; three

triceps [TRY-seps] having three heads or subdivisions

triceps brachii muscle [TRY-seps BRAY-kee-eye MUS-sel] muscle on the dorsal surface of the humerus that extends the forearm when flexed

trichomycosis [trik-oh-migh-KOH-sis] fungal hair disease

trichotillomania [TRIK-oh-TIL-oh-MAY-nee-ah] repetitive pulling out of hair from the head

tricuspid atresia [try-KUS-pid ah-TREE-see-ah] congenital absence of the tricuspid valve of the heart

tricuspid valve [try-KUS-pid valv] a structure of the heart that allows blood to flow in one direction from the right atrium to the right ventricle

trigeminal neuralgia [trye-JEM-ih-nul new-RHAL-juh] pain in one or more branches of cranial nerve V

trigeminy [try-JEM-ih-nee] occurrence of events in groups of three, especially three rapid heartbeats

triglyceride [try-GLIS-er-yd] a simple fat molecule consisting of three molecules of fatty acids and glycerol; they combine with lipoproteins in the blood and are stored in body tissues as fat

triiodothyronine (T3) [tri-eye-oh-doh-THY-roh-neen] one of the hormones secreted by the thyroid gland

-tripsy [trip-see] *suffix*; to crush

-trophy [tro-fee] *suffix*; to nourish or develop

troponin I [TRO-po-nin wun] a highly sensitive and specific indicator of recent cardiac muscle damage

trousseau sign [true-SOH sighn] carpal tetany elicited when the brachial or forearm region is compressed due to hypocalcemia

true ribs [TRU ribz] the first seven pairs of curved bones that form the upper thoracic cage and are individually attached by cartilage to the sternum

true vocal cords [tru voh-KAL kordz] lower folds of the larynx that produce sound by vibrating as air moves out of the lungs

truncus arteriosus [TRUN-kus ar-tee-ree-OH-sis] heart malformation in which a single large vessel empties both ventricles, causing cyanosis to develop soon after birth with severe congestive heart failure, dyspnea, retractions, fatigue, polycythemia, clubbing, increased pulse pressure, bounding peripheral pulses, and cardiomegaly

truss [TRUHS] an externally applied device used to apply pressure to a hernia to prevent it from enlarging or protruding

tubal ligation [TU-bal lye-GAY-shun] female sterilization by surgical excision and closure of the fallopian tube so that conception cannot occur

tubercles [TOO-ber-klz] small lesions of inflammation associated with tuberculosis

tuberculosis [too-BER-kyoo-LOH-sis] a chronic granulomatous infection caused by an acid-fast bacillus, *Mycobacterium tuberculosis*

tubule [TOO-byool] a series of compartmentalized, small tubes that collect or transport substances in bodily organs

tumescence [tyoo-MES-ens] condition of being swollen or with edema

tumor suppressor genes [TOO-mor soo-PRES-sor jeenz] genetic material that controls the growth of cells, decreasing the effects of cancer-producing stimuli

tunica [TOO-ni-kah] fibro-elastic tissue that covers or coats tubular structures such as blood or lymph vessels

tunica externa [TOO-ni-kah ecks-TUR-nah] outermost layer of connective tissue covering an organ or structure that is not covered by a serosa

tunica media [TOO-ni-kah MEE-dee-ah] middle layer of the coating of a blood or lymph vessel; comprised of smooth muscle

turbidimetry [tur-bih-DIM-eh-tree] measurement of the relative cloudiness of a solution, such as urine, in which the amount of light able to pass through the substance is quantified by using a spectrophotometer

turbinate [TER-bin-ayt] coil-like structures, one on each side of the nasal septum, that act as barriers to divide and slow the passage of inhaled air so that it can pick up warmth and moisture

turgor [TUR-gur] normal skin tension

Turner's syndrome [TUR-nerz SIN-drom] a chromosomal anomaly occurring in approximately 1 in 3,000 births due to the absence of one X chromosome; characterized by webbing of neck skin, cardiovascular abnormalities, ovarian failure, shield-shaped chest, and underdevelopment of breast, uterus, and vagina

tussis [TUS-is] coughing

tympani [tym-PAN-ee] loud, high-pitched sounds similar to a drum, usually heard over an air-filled stomach

tympanic membrane [tym-PAN-ik MEM-brayn] a structure that is a thick but pliable tissue that registers sound and causes vibrations to be transmitted to the inner ear; also known as the eardrum

tympanogram [tim-PAN-oh-gram] a graphic record of the movement of the tympanic membrane in response to air-pressure changes in the external auditory canal

tympanometry [TIM-pah-NAWM-eh-tree] a hearing test that measures the ability of the tympanic membrane in the ear to move in response to air pressure (rather than sound)

tympanoplasty [tim-pah-no-PLAS-tee] surgical reconstruction of a ruptured tympanic membrane

tympanotomy tubes [tym-pan-AWT-oh-mee toobz] surgical insertion of small Teflon tubes in the tympanic membrane to equalize pressure, promote fluid drainage, and ventilate the middle ear

Tzanck [ZANK] a differential skin test using Giemsa stain with microscopic examination

U

-ula [uhle-uh] *suffix*; small

ulcer [UL-sur] slow-healing sore on the surface of an organ or tissue resulting from tissue necrosis

ulcerative colitis [UL-ser-ah-tiv koh-LY-tis] an inflammatory disease of the ileum and colon with inflammation followed by areas of normal mucosa known as enteritis; the disease affects the colon and rectum; treatment may involve steroids and removal of affected segments of intestine

ulcerative keratitis [UL-ser-ah-tiv KER-ah-ty-tis] erosion of the cornea

-ule [uhle] *suffix*; small

ulna [UL-nah] forearm bone located along the little-finger side of the lower arm

ulnar drift [UL-nar drift] alteration in the position of the metacarpophalangeal joints where the fingers curve toward the ulnar bone of the forearm; results from rheumatoid arthritis

ultra- [ul-trah] *prefix*; extreme, beyond, or disproportionate

ultrasonogram [ul-trah-SON-oh-gram] use of sound waves to assess the body structures and create computerized images for study

ultrasound [UL-trah-sownd] noninvasive procedure that generates images via computer analysis to assess blood-flow velocity, direction, and occlusions; uses a transducer, which is placed over the blood vessel, and a computer, which analyzes the echoes for aberrations

umbilical cord [um-BIL-ih-kul kord] a vascular structure attaching the fetus to the placenta in utero

umbilicate [um-BIL-ih-KAYT] having the appearance of being pitted or indented; shaped like an umbilicus; used to describe some skin conditions

umbilicus [um-bih-LIE-kus] depressed point on the surface of the abdomen where the umbilical cord was formerly attached

uni- [yoo-nee] *prefix*; one, singular

unigravida [yoo-nee-GRAV-ih-da] a woman who is pregnant for the first time

unilateral [yoo-nih-LAT-er-ahl] confined to one side

universal precautions [yoo-nih-VER-sal pre-KAW-shuns] standard measures to prevent exposure to blood-borne pathogens

Unna's boot [YOO-naz boot] a dressing applied to stasis ulcers of the lower leg using layers of gauze and a mixture of zinc oxide in a glycogelatin base

unremarkable [un-re-MARK-uh-bull] no significance or information worth noting, all normal findings

upper gastrointestinal series (UGI) [UP-err gas-troh-en-TES-tih-nal SEER-eez] study of the esophagus, stomach, and sometimes small bowel after swallowing barium sulfate solution

uraniscoplasty [yoo-rayn-is-KOH-plas-tee] surgical repair of a cleft palate

uraniscus [yoo-ran-IS-kus] palate or roof of the mouth

uranoplegia [yoo-rah-noh-PLEE-jee-ah] paralysis of the soft palate of the mouth

uremia [yoo-REE-mee-ah] excessive urea and nitrogenous wastes in the blood

uremic frost [yoo-REE-mik frawst] skin appears powdery as a result of severe uremia due to dermal deposits of urea and uric acid salt

ureter [YOO-reh-tur] one of two small tubes that drain urine from the kidneys to the bladder

ureteritis [yoo-ree-ter-EYE-tis] inflammation of the ureter

ureterocystostomy [yoo-ree-tur-oh-SIS-TOS-tuh-mee] surgical connection made between the ureter and the bladder

urethra [yoo-REE-thra] the short vessel used for the purpose of eliminating or passing urine

urethritis [yoo-ree-THRIGH-tis] inflammation of the urethra caused by infection or mechanical irritation associated with a stone

urethroplasty [yoo-REE-throh-PLAS-tee] surgical procedure that involves plastic surgery to reposition the urethra; used to correct congenital hypospadias or epispadias

-uria [yoo-ree-ah] *suffix*; pertaining to urine or urination

uric acid [YOO-rik AS-id] an end product of protein metabolism that is present in measurable quantities and ultimately excreted in urine

uricosuria [yoo-ri-koh-SOO-ree-ah] presence of abnormal amounts of uric acid in the urine

urinalysis [yoo-ri-NAL-ih-sis] examination of the urine

urinary sand [YOOR-ih-nair-ee sand] passage of multiple minute, non-obstructing calculous particles in the urine following nephrolithiasis

urinary tract [YOOR-ih-nair-ee trakt] structures leading from the urinary pelvis of the kidney, ureters, and bladder to the urethra

urine amylase test [YOOR-un AM-il-ace] test measuring pancreatic urine levels of amylase

urine ketosteroid tests [YOOR-un kee-toh-STEER-oid tests] analyses of urine to detect androgen metabolites

urine turbidity [YOOR-in tur-BID-ih-tee] refers to the clarity of liquid excreted by the kidney

urinophil [YOO-rih-noh-fil] organisms such as bacteria that thrive in the urinary bladder or urine

urochrome [YOOR-oh-krome] yellow pigment found in urine

urodynia [yoo-roh-DIN-ee-ah] painful urination; often associated with urinary tract infection

urologist [yoo-RAWL-oh-ist] a licensed physician who specializes in the treatment of disorders of the urinary tract

urostomy [yur-OS-toh-mee] diversion of urine into a surgically created opening in the abdominal wall so that urine drains continually into an attached appliance or bag.

urticaria [ur-tih-KAR-ee-ah] hives marked by redness and swelling wheals

-us [us] *suffix*; structure or thing

uterine cavity [YOO-ter-in KAV-ih-tee] hollow space within the uterus

uterine fibroids [YOO-ter-in FYE-broidz] benign muscle tumor of the uterus; also known as fibroids, aromas, myomas, leiomyoma, or fibromyomas

uterine inertia [YOO-ter-in in-ER-shah] lack of effective contractions during labor

uterine lining [YOO-ter-in LYN-ing] endometrial tissue

uterine prolapse [YOO-ter-in PRO-laps] protrusion or displacement of the uterus through the vaginal canal; assigned stages one to three depending on how far into the vaginal canal the uterus has fallen

uterovesical [YOO-ter-oh-VES-ik-ahl] pertaining to the uterus and bladder

uterus [YOO-ter-us] hollow muscular organ of the female reproductive tract where a fertilized ovum implants and develops into a fetus

uveal tract [YOO-vee-ahl TRAKT] collective term for the ciliary body of the eye; also known as the uvea

uvula [YOO-voo-lah] the fleshy hanging part of the soft palate that activates the gag reflex when stimulated

uvulopalatopharyngoplasty [YOO-voo-lo-PAL-ah-toh-FAIR-in-go-plas-tee] plastic surgical procedure to remove excess soft palate, uvula, and other structures of the throat to resolve sleep apnea and intractable snoring

V

vaccination [VAK-sih-NAY-shun] medical procedure that injects a vaccine into the body

vaccine [vak-SEEN] killed or attenuated bacterial or viral cells or cell fragments used to trigger the production of antibodies and memory B lymphocytes specific to that pathogen; routinely used to prevent diseases; also known as immunization

vagal nerve stimulation [VAY-gal nerv stim-yoo-LAY-shun] treatment of intractable seizure disorder where electrical impulses are delivered in 30-second segments every five minutes by a device implanted in the anterior wall

vagina [vah-JYN-ah] the musculomembranous tube that connects the cervix uteri and the vulva

vaginomycosis [VAJ-in-oh-migh-KOH-sis] fungal infection of the vagina

vagolysis [vay-go-LY-sis] surgical destruction of the vagus (X) nerve interrupting the impulses transmitted to the stomach and intestines

valgus [VAL-gus] structural deformation of being bent or turned outward; most often used to describe extremities

Valsalva maneuver [val-SAHL-vuh ma-NEW-vur] forced expiratory effort

valvuloplasty [VALV-yoo-loh-PLAS-tee] dilation of a heart valve to relieve stenosis by balloon dilatation during cardiac catheterization or surgery

vanillylmandelic acid [VAN-ih-lil-man-DEL-ik AS-id] the urinary metabolite that is elevated in patients with pheochromocytoma

vaporizer [VAY-por-iz-er] a device for changing liquid medications to a gaseous state for the purpose of inhalation

varicocelectomy [VAR-ih-koh-see-LEK-toh-mee] surgical excision of the scrotal sac and dilated veins

varicose [VAR-ih-kose] veins that are knotted or swollen; they often occur in the lower legs and esophagus due to defective vein valves; plural is varix

varus [VAR-us] condition in which the hind foot turns inward; usually associated with clubfoot

vasa recta [VAH-sa REK-tah] capillary network of a nephron in the kidney

vasa vasorum [VAH-sa vah-SOH-rum] minute blood vessels in the walls of larger arteries and veins

vascular aneurysm [VAS-kew-lur AN-yoo-riz-um] sac-shaped outward bulge on an artery

vascular murmur [VAS-kew-lur MUR-mur] turbulent blood flow due to incomplete closure of heart

vascular stasis [VAS-kyoo-lar STA-sis] pooling of blood in the periphery

vascular stent [VAS-kyoo-lar stent] intravascular insertion of a tubular meshwork to keep an artery open

vascularization] [VAS-kyoo-lar-eye-ZAY-shun] development of new blood vessels in tissue such as the myocardium

vasectomy [vas-EK-toh-mee] surgical procedure involving bilateral surgical removal of part of the vas deferens for the purpose of sterilization

vasoconstriction [vays-oh-kon-STRIK-shun] decrease in the diameter of a blood vessel

vasodilators [vayz-oh-dye-LAY-tors] drugs that widen blood vessels, decreasing blood pressure

vastus intermedius muscle [VAS-tus in-tur-MEE-dee-us MUS-sel] muscle of the anterior thigh covering the femoral shaft, situated between the vastus lateralis and vastus medialis; it functions to extends the lower leg

vastus lateralis muscle [VAS-tus lat-ur-AL-is MUS-sel] largest muscle of the anterior lateral aspect of the femoral shaft that extends the lower leg; often used for injection site

vastus medialis muscle [VAS-tus mee-dee-AL-is MUS-sel] muscle of the anterior thigh situated on the interior aspect of the femoral shaft that extends the lower leg

vein sclerosing [vayn skle-ROWS-ing] injection of a hypertonic solution, causing the vein to harden and eventually atrophy

vein stripping [vayn STRIP-ing] surgical removal of a vein after ligation of varicose veins

veins [VAYNZ] vessels carrying blood toward the heart

venipuncture [VEN-ih-punk-chur] piercing a venous blood vessel for the purpose of obtaining a blood sample

venography [vee-NOG-rah-fee] x-ray examination of the veins after injection of dye that absorbs the x-rays

venostasis [vee-noh-STAY-sis] method of reducing the amount of blood returning to the heart by compression of veins in the periphery

ventilator [VEN-tih-lay-tor] any of several devices used in respiratory therapy to provide assisted respiration and intensive positive-pressure breathing

ventral [VEN-tral] front

-ventral [ven-tral] *suffix*; pertaining to the stomach or abdominal area

ventral phimosis [VEN-tral figh-MOH-sis] stenosis of the penis prepuce

ventral ramus [VEN-tral RAY-mus] a branch of the spinal nerve that supplies nervous impulses to the lateral portions of the body wall, ribs, and perineum

ventral root [VEN-tral root] the nerve tract that connects the spinal cord to motor neurons and transmits impulses to muscles, producing movement

ventricle [VEN-trih-kel] a space or chamber in an organ; for example, the lower chambers of the heart

ventricular assist device [ven-TRIK-yoo-lar ah-SIST dee-VYS] a mechanical device that supports or replaces the function of the right or left ventricle of the heart in clients with severely diseased or nonfunctioning heart muscle

ventricular fibrillation [ven-TRIK-yoo-lar fib-ril-LAY-shun] rapid but ineffective movements of the ventricles of the heart that replace coordinated contractions, resulting in grossly diminished cardiac output

ventricular hypertrophy [ven-TRIK-yoo-lar hy-PER-troh-fee] pathological enlargement of the ventricles of the heart; often associated with valve disease, heart failure, or hypertension

ventricular septal defect [ven-TRIK-yoo-lur SEP-tul DEE-fekt] an abnormal opening between the ventricles, allowing blood to shunt back and forth

ventriculoperitoneal shunt [ven-TRIK-yoo-loh-per-it-oh-NEE-al shunt] surgical placement of tubing in the cerebral ventricle, tube has one-way valves to drain excess cerebrospinal fluid from the brain to treat hydrocephalus

venules [VAYN-yoolz] smallest branches of veins

vermiform appendix [VER-mih-form ah-PEN-diks] a wormlike intestinal diverticulum located at the end of the cecum and terminating in a blind extremity

vermilion border [ver-MIL-yon BOR-dur] the pink-red border around the lips

vermis [VUR-mis] lobe of the cerebellum between the two hemispheres

verruca vulgaris [ver-ROO-kuh vul-GAIR-us] common wart; caused by viral infection of the skin

vertebrae [VER-teh-bree] individual bones of the spinal column

vertebral column [VER-teh-bral KOL-um] collective name for the cervical, thoracic, lumbar and sacral bones of the dorsal spine

vertical transmission [VER-tih-cal trans-MIH-shun] passage of disease from the mother to the fetus during the period of pregnancy

vertigo [VER-tih-goh] dizziness while not moving, and ringing in the ears in quiet environments

vesical [VES-ih-kal] pertaining to the urinary bladder

vesicles [VES-ih-kuls] blisters that leak fluid

vesicoureteral reflux [VEZ-ih-koh-yoo-REE-ter-al REE-fluks] retrograde flow of urine from the bladder into the ureter

vesicovaginal fistula [ves-ih-koh-VA-jin-ahl FIS-tyoo-lah] an abnormal opening between the bladder and vagina

vestibule [VES-tih-byool] chamber of the inner ear

vibices [VYE-bi-seez] bruising in a linear pattern on the skin

villi [VILL-eye] projections from the surface of the gastric mucosa

viral hepatitis [VYE-ral hep-ah-TYE-tis] inflammation of the liver due to a viral infection

viral load [VYE-ral lohd] plasma measurement of viral RNA, usually done in serial fashion with human immunodeficiency disorder

virilism [VIR-il-izm] development of male secondary sex characteristics in a female

virulent [VIR-yoo-lens] highly toxic or intense disease-producing quality of a pathogen

viscera [VIS-er-ah] all of the internal organs of the various body cavities

visceral muscle [VIS-er-al MUS-sel] smooth muscle of the internal organs

visceral pericardium [VIS-eh-ral perr-ih-KAHR-dee-um] layer directly on the outside of the heart muscle

viscid [VIS-kid] a thick and sticky substance; for example, mucus secretions

viscosity [vis-KAWS-ih-tee] the resistance of a substance to change in shape or flow due to molecular cohesion; most often applied to liquids

visual cortex [VIZH-yoo-ahl KOR-teks] areas in the right and left occipital lobes of the brain that merge images from both eyes to create a single image that is right side up and in its original horizontal direction

vital capacity (VC) [VYE-tal kah-PAS-ih-tee] the maximum volume of air that can be exhaled following the deepest inhalation; calculated as: tidal volume + inspiratory reserve volume + expiratory reserve volume; average value = 4,500 cc

vital signs [VYE-tal sighns] objective measures of key body parameters, such as temperature, breathing rate, pulse, and blood pressure

vitiligo [vit-ih-LYE-go] skin disease characterized by patches without pigmentation

vitrectomy [vih-TREK-toh-mee] removing the vitreous humor and replacing it with a synthetic substitute

vitreous humor [VIT-ree-us HYOO-mor] clear, gel-like substance that fills the posterior cavity of the eye

vocal fremitus [VOL-kal FREM-ih-tus] palpable vibration in the chest wall produced by voice sounds due to consolidates or congestion

voiding cystourethrography [VOY-ding SIS-toh-YOO-ree-THRAWG-rah-fee] radiographic examination of the bladder before, during, and after voiding

voluntary muscle [VAWL-un-tar-ee MUS-sel] skeletal muscles that contract or relax in response to conscious thought

volvulus [VOLV-yoo-lus] twisting of a loop of intestine around itself or around another segment of bowel, causing obstruction

vomer [VOH-mer] a narrow wafer of bone that forms the inferior part of the nasal septum that continues posteriorly to the cranium, where it joins the sphenoid bone

vomicose [VOM-ih-kose] condition of having many ulcers with purulent drainage

vomitus [VOHM-ih-tus] expelled food or chyme

vulvar carcinoma [VUL-var kar-sin-OH-mah] malignant neoplasm of the vulva, most often squamous cell type, with the greatest incidence in women ages 65–70 years

vulvorectal [vul-voh-REK-tal] pertaining to the vulva and rectal area

W

wave lithotripsy [wayv lith-oh-TRIP-see] fragmentation of stones using ultrasound short waves so that the pulverized pieces can pass naturally

Weber test for hearing [WEH-ber TEST for HEER-ing] assessment of bone conduction of sound by placing a vibrating tuning fork at the midpoint of the forehead to determine if sound is heard equally in both ears

Wernicke's aphasia [VER-nih-keez ah-FAY-zee-uh] deficit in ability to comprehend sounds or written words due to damage to the temporal lobe by trauma or stroke

Wernicke's encephalopathy [VER-nih-keez en-sef-ah-LOP-ah-thee] brain damage with gross short-term memory disruption due to chronic alcoholism and thiamine deficiency

wet gangrene [wet GANG-green] ischemia and necrosis of tissue with bacterial infection causing cellulitis in adjacent tissues

wheal [WHEEL] swellings in specific skin areas

wheezes [WHEE zes] audible whistling breath sound often associated with asthma or airway constriction

white matter [whyt MAT-ter] the tissue of the central nervous system consisting mainly of myelinated nerve fibers

Wilms tumor [VILMS tu-mor] a rapidly developing malignant neoplasm of the kidney of unknown etiology, seen in infants and children before age five; it may be treated with surgery, radiation, or chemotherapy

windowing [WIN-dow-ing] to cut a hole in a cast or other material to relieve pressure on the skin or a bony prominence

withdrawal syndrome [with-DRAWL SIN-drom] uncomfortable physical symptoms that occur when use of a sedative, pain drug, or illegal narcotic is stopped suddenly in a patient who is physically tolerant

word salad [word SAL-ad] speech that includes a jumble of seemingly unrelated words; often associated with thought disorders such as schizophrenia

X

xanthoma [zan-THO-muh] fat-filled cells in subcutaneous tissue

xeno- [zee-noh] *prefix*; strange or odd

xenograft [ZEN-oh-graft] tissue graft from a distant species

xeroderma [zeer-oh-DUR-mah] extremely dry skin

xeroderma pigmentosum [zeer-oh-DUR-mah pig-men-TOH-sum] abnormal skin-thickening caused by viral infection

xerophthalmia [ZEER-opf-THAL-mee-ah] insufficient production of tears because of eye irritation, associated aging process, or an ectropion of the eyelid

x-rays [EKS-rayz] use of electromagnetic radiation to penetrate body parts and produce images used for diagnosis and treatment of a wide variety of conditions

xyphoid process [ZY-foyd PRAW-sess] the small tip at the inferior end of the sternum

Y

-y [ee] *suffix*; condition or process

Yankauer suction catheter [YAWN-kur SUK-shun KATH-eh-ter] a rigid, plastic-tipped device used to aspirate secretions from the mouth and throat

yolk sack [yohk sak] embryonic membranous tissue that produces the first red blood cell of the embryo

Z

Zollinger-Ellison syndrome [ZOL-in-jer EL-ih-sun SIN-drom] hypersecretion of gastric acid and formation of gastric ulcers; associated with nonbeta cell tumors of the pancreatic isles

zoonosis [zoh-oh-NO-sis] spread of disease from animals to humans

Z-plasty [zee-PLAS-tee] use of a Z-shaped surgical incision to reduce tension on a scar produced by normal movement of a body part

z-track method [ZEE-trak METH-od] a technique of administering an intramuscular injection that prevents the fluid from seeping out of the site by pulling the skin tightly to one side, administering the injection, removing the needle, then allowing the skin to slide back into the normal position

zygomatic bones [ZY-goh-mah-tik bohnz] facial bones that form the lateral edges of the eye sockets and cheekbones

zygomaticus muscle [zye-goh-MAT-ih-kus MUS-sel] the facial muscle that draws the corner of the mouth upward and outward

zygote [ZYE gote] a fertilized ovum

Resource Lists

2

➤ RESOURCE CATEGORY 1: ANATOMY/PHYSIOLOGY

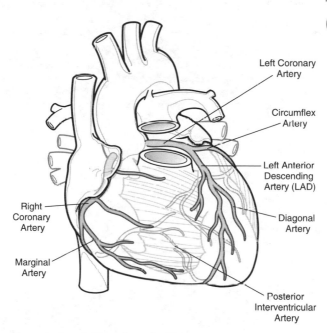

Left Coronary Artery

Circumflex Artery

Left Anterior Descending Artery (LAD)

Diagonal Artery

Right Coronary Artery

Marginal Artery

Posterior Interventricular Artery

Figure 1: Arterial Supply to the Heart

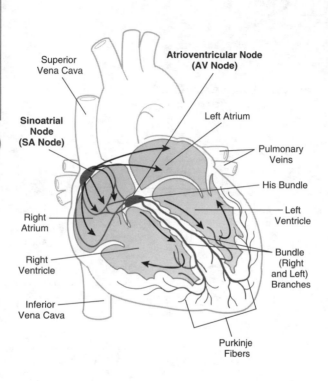

Figure 2: Cardiac Conduction System

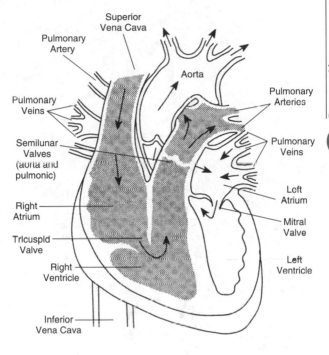

Figure 3: Cardiovascular System, Heart

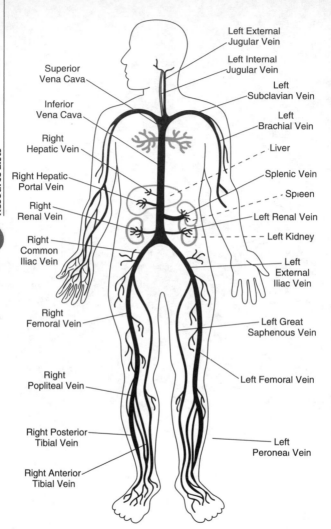

Figure 4: Cardiovascular System, Major Veins

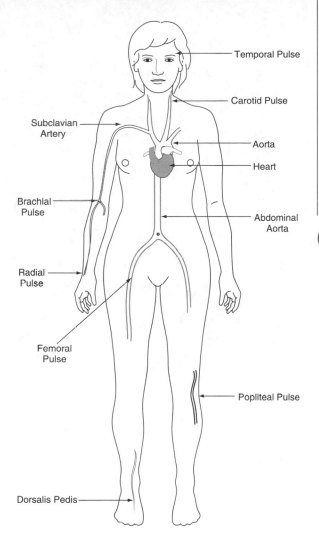

Temporal Pulse

Carotid Pulse

Subclavian Artery

Aorta

Heart

Brachial Pulse

Abdominal Aorta

Radial Pulse

Femoral Pulse

Popliteal Pulse

Dorsalis Pedis

Figure 5: Cardiovascular System, Pulse Points

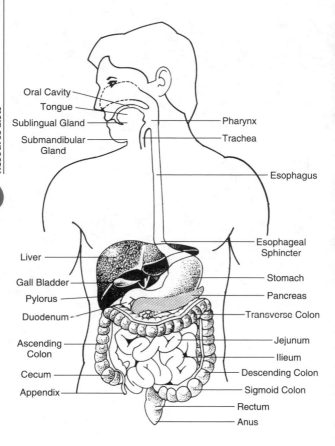

Oral Cavity
Tongue
Sublingual Gland
Submandibular Gland
Pharynx
Trachea
Esophagus
Esophageal Sphincter
Liver
Gall Bladder
Pylorus
Duodenum
Ascending Colon
Cecum
Appendix
Stomach
Pancreas
Transverse Colon
Jejunum
Ilieum
Descending Colon
Sigmoid Colon
Rectum
Anus

Figure 6: Digestive System

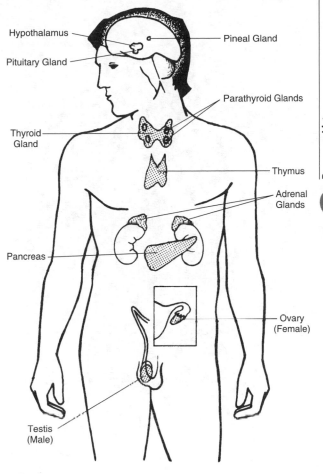

Hypothalamus

Pituitary Gland

Pineal Gland

Parathyroid Glands

Thyroid Gland

Thymus

Adrenal Glands

Pancreas

Ovary (Female)

Testis (Male)

Figure 7: Endocrine System

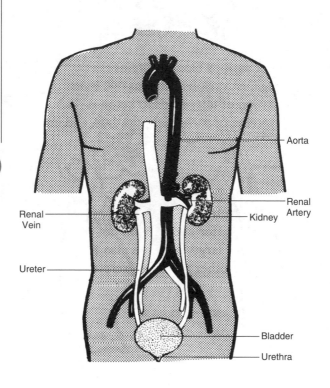

Figure 8: Excretory System

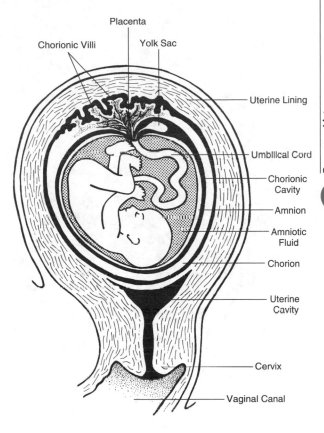

Chorionic Villi

Placenta

Yolk Sac

Uterine Lining

Umbilical Cord

Chorionic Cavity

Amnion

Amniotic Fluid

Chorion

Uterine Cavity

Cervix

Vaginal Canal

Figure 9: Human Fetus

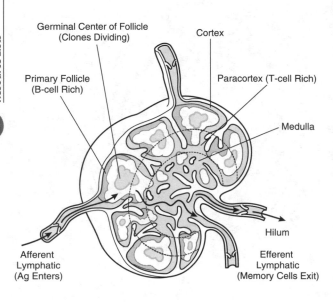

Figure 10: Lymph Node

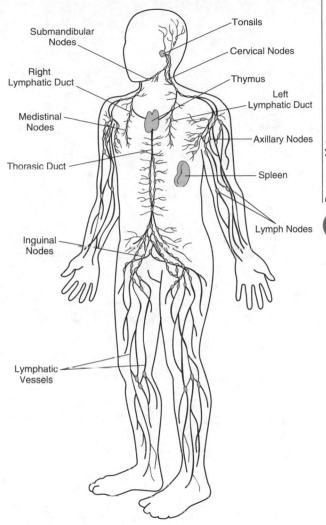

Figure 11: Lymphatic System

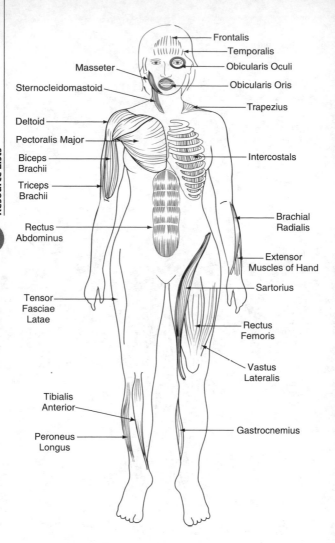

Figure 12: Muscles, Anterior

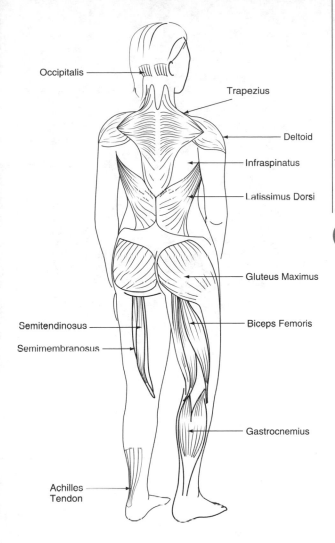

Occipitalis

Trapezius

Deltoid

Infraspinatus

Latissimus Dorsi

Gluteus Maximus

Semitendinosus

Biceps Femoris

Semimembranosus

Gastrocnemius

Achilles Tendon

Figure 13: Muscles, Posterior

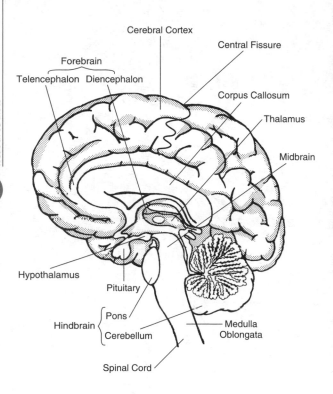

Figure 14: Nervous System, Brain

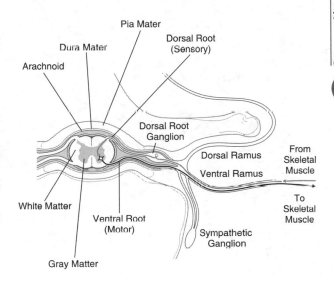

Figure 15: Nervous System, Cross-Section of Spinal Cord and the Components of a Spinal Nerve

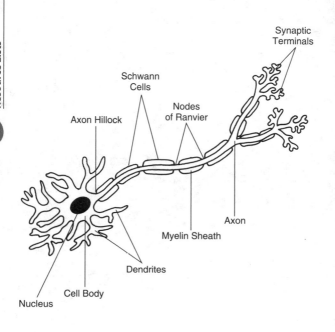

Figure 16: Nervous System, Neuron

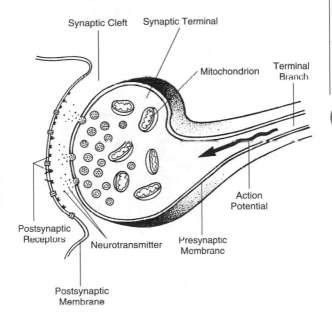

Figure 17: Nervous System, Synapse

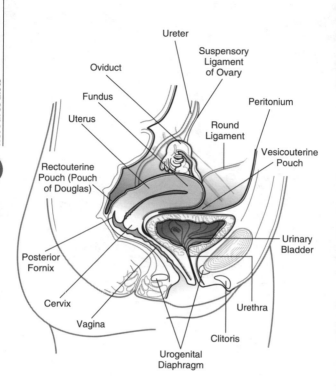

Ureter

Suspensory
Ligament
of Ovary

Oviduct

Peritonium

Fundus

Round
Ligament

Uterus

Vesicouterine
Pouch

Rectouterine
Pouch (Pouch
of Douglas)

Urinary
Bladder

Posterior
Fornix

Urethra

Cervix

Clitoris

Vagina

Urogenital
Diaphragm

Figure 18: Reproductive System, Female

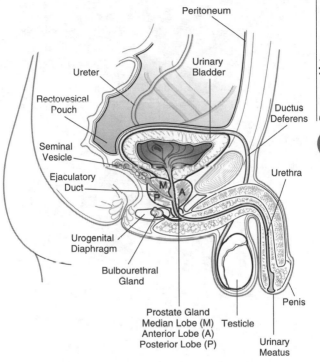

Peritoneum

Ureter

Urinary Bladder

Rectovesical Pouch

Ductus Deferens

Seminal Vesicle

Ejaculatory Duct

Urethra

Urogenital Diaphragm

Bulbourethral Gland

Prostate Gland
Median Lobe (M)
Anterior Lobe (A)
Posterior Lobe (P)

Testicle

Penis

Urinary Meatus

Figure 19: Reproductive System, Male

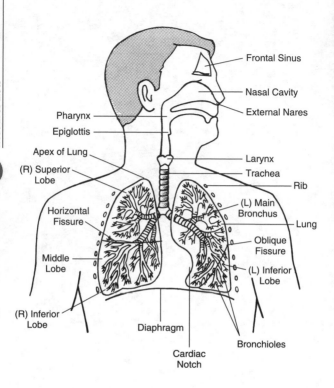

Figure 20: Respiratory System

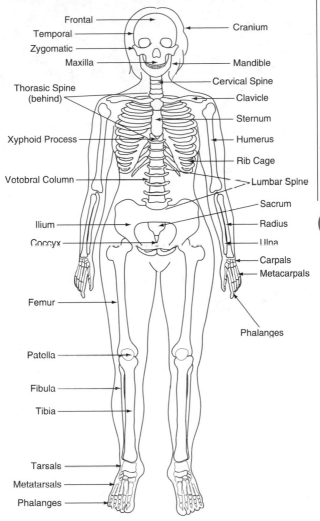

Figure 21: Skeletal System, Bones

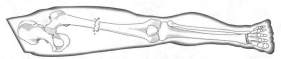

A. Transverse: Break across Entire Cross-Section of Bone

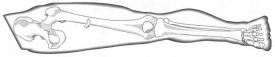

B. Incomplete: Break through Portion of Bone

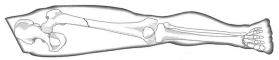

C. Closed: No External Communication

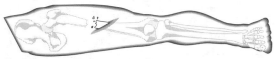

D. Compound: Extends through Skin

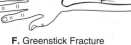

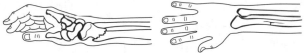

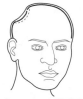

E. Colles Fracture

F. Greenstick Fracture

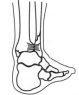

G. Depressed Skull Fracture

H. Pott's Fracture

Figure 22: Skeletal System, Fractures

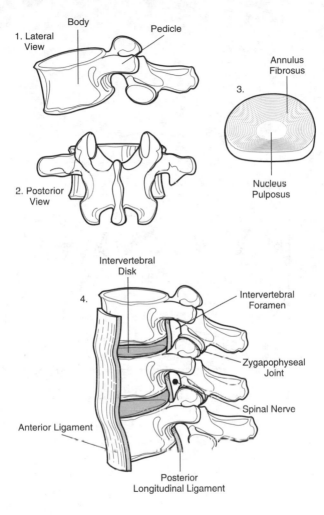

Figure 23: Skeletal System, Intervertebral Foramen

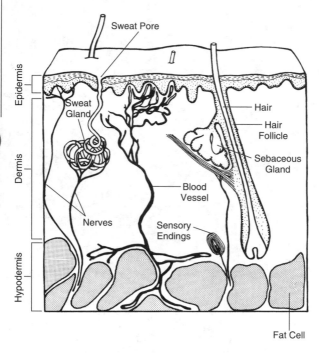

Figure 24: Skin

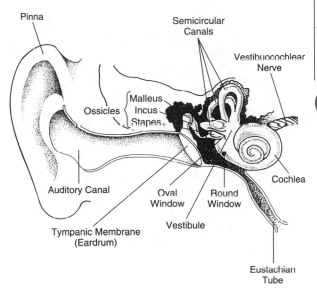

Figure 25: Special Sense Organs, Ear

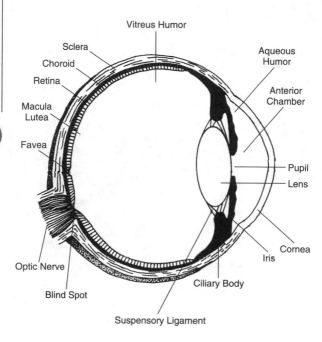

Figure 26: Special Sense Organs, Eye

General Pathology

Neurological Disorders

acetylcholine
agnosia
agraphia
Alzheimer's disease
amyotrophic lateral sclerosis
aphagia
aphasia
apraxia
Asperger's disorder
athetosis
autism
Babinski sign
Bell's palsy
cataplexy
catastrophic reaction
cerebral palsy
circumstantiality
cognition
concussion

coup-contre coup
delirium
delirium tremens
dementia
encephalitis
Erb palsy
Huntington chorea
hydrocephalus
Lewy body dementia
multi-infarct dementia
multiple sclerosis
myasthenia gravis
progressive supranuclear
   palsy
punch drunk syndrome
seizure
tonic-clonic movements
Wernicke syndrome

Cancer

adenocarcinoma
antineoplastics
astrocytoma
basal cell carcinoma
chemotherapy
Cheyne-Stokes respirations

dyscrasia
ependymoma
Ewing's sarcoma
hepatoma
inguinodynia
lymphadenopathy

lymphangioma
lymphoma
medulloblastoma
metastasize
myelogenous leukemia
neoplasm
neoplastic
nephroblastoma
osteosarcoma

palliative care
patient-controlled analgesia
polyadenoma
precancerous
radiation therapy
rhabdomyosarcoma
squamous cell carcinoma
T cells
tumor suppressor genes

COPD

antitussives
arterial blood gases
bronchodilator
circumoral cyanosis
clubbing of fingers
cough
cyanosis
effusion
emphysema
empyema
endotoxin
endotracheal intubation
epinephrine
expectorate
expiratory reserve volume

extubation
hemoptysis
hypercapnia
hypoglycemia
incentive spirometry
intercostal retractions
mucolytic
mucopurulent
nebulizer
perfusion
pulse oximeter
sepsis
tracheobronchial suction
vaporizer
vocal fremitus

Respiratory Diseases

acute respiratory distress
    syndrome
antihistamines
aspiration pneumonia
assist-control ventilation
asthma

atelectasis
bag-valve-mask
bronchial asthma
bronchiectasis
bronchitis
bronchodilators

bronchopneumonia
bronchospasm
chest physiotherapy
controlled mandatory
    ventilation
empyema
hyaline membrane disease
hyperresonance
mechanical ventilation
oligopnea

peak expiratory flow
pleural effusion
pleuralgia
pneumocentesis
pneumoconiosis
Pneumocystis carinii
pneumonia
pneumothorax
pulmonary atresio
pyothorax

Diabetes

alkalosis
amylase
antidiabetic drugs
atonic bladder
diabetes insipidus
diabetes mellitus
diabetes mellitus, type I
diabetes mellitus, type II
diabetes neuropathy
diabetic ketoacidosis
diabetic retinopathy
fructosuria
glucagon
glucometer
glucosuria
glycohemoglobin

glycosylated hemoglobin
hyperinsulinism
hypoglycemia
hyposecretion
insulin resistance
insulin shock
ketonuria
metabolic syndrome
neurogenic bladder
oral antidiabetic
pancreas
pancreatic islets
pancreatography
polydipsia
retinopathy

Heart Disease

aberrant conduction
angiospasm
angiostenosis
aortalgia

aortic stenosis
asynchronous pacing
atherosclerotic plaque
atrial ectopic beats

atrial fibrillation
atrial septal defect
cardiomyopathy
cardioplegia
cardioversion
carotid sinus syndrome
coarctation of the aorta
congestive heart disease
congestive heart failure
cor pulmonale
coronary bypass
digitalization
dissecting aneurysm
ejection murmur
endopericarditis
hyperlipidemia
implanted cardioverter
   defibrillator

intermittent claudication
mitral valve prolapse
myocardial infarction
myocarditis
neoplastic heart syndrome
pacing catheter
phlebothrombosis
premature atrial contractions
pulmonic stenosis
sinus tachycardia
supraventricular tachycardia
tissue plasminogen
   activator
tricuspid atresia
vascular stent
ventricular fibrillation
ventricular hypertrophy

Parkinson's Disease

anosmia
anticholinergics
astasia
asterixis
asthenia
ataxia
bradykinesia
bradyphrasia
cerebellar gait
cogwheeling
dopamine
dyskinesia
dysphagia
dysphonia
dystonia

extrapyramidal side effects
galt apraxia
hypokinetic dysarthria
myoclonus
neuroleptic
oculogyric crisis
pallidotomy
Parkinson facies
rigidity
sialorrhea
somnolent
tardive dyskinesia
torpid
tremor

Sexually Transmitted Diseases

acquired immunodeficiency syndrome (AIDS)
amebiasis
bacterial vaginosis
balanitis
chancroid
Chlamydia trachomatis
colposcope
condyloma acuminatum
cryptosporidiosis
cystitis
cytomegalovirus
giardiasis
gonorrhea
hepatitus A
hepatitis B
hepatitis C
herpes simplex
human papilloma virus
Kaposi's sarcoma
lymphogranuloma venereum
molluscum contagiosum
pelvic inflammatory disease
proctocolitis
protease inhibitor drugs
scabies
sexually transmitted disease
syphilis
viral load
vulvar carcinoma

Stroke

anisocoria
aphagia
aphasia
asaphia
atony
atrophy
bradyglossia
cerebral angiography
cerebral edema
cerebral perfusion pressure
cerebrovascular accident
coma
contracture
decerebrate rigidity
dystonia
enteral nutrition
flaccid
Glasgow coma scale
hemianopia
hemiparesis
hemiplegia
hemorrhagic stroke
ischemic stroke
monoplegia
paralysis
paresthesia
phlebosclerosis
phrenoplegia
thrombolytic therapy
transient ischemic attack

Procedures

Diagnostic

air-puff tonometry
alanine aminotransferase
    test
angiogram
arthrogram
barium enema
biopsy
bone densitometry
bone marrow aspiration
cardiac catheterization
cardiac scan
colposcopy
computerized axial
    tomography
culdocentesis
digital subtraction
    angiography
dilated funduscopy
echocardiogram

electrocardiogram
electroencephalograph
endoscopic retrograde
    cholangiopancreatography
fluorescein angiography
fluoroscopy
lumbar puncture
magnetic resonance
    imaging
pulmonary function tests
pulmonary ventilation scan
radioactive iodine uptake
    test
radionuclide scan
scintigraphy
single-photon emission
    computed tomography
thyroid scan
voiding cystourethrography

Surgical

adrenalectomy
angioplasty
appendectomy
bladder neck suspension
cardiopulmonary bypass graft
cecocolopexy
chondrectomy
colpoperineoplasty
craniotomy
cystostomy

dacryocystorhinostomy
endarterectomy
enterocolectomy
ganglionectomy
gastrectomy
hemicolectomy
hysterectomy
ileotomy
laryngectomy
laryngotracheotomy

laser-assisted in situ
  keratomileusis
lymphangioplasty
myringotomy
orchidoplasty
polypectomy
prostatectomy
radical neck dissection
rhizotomy

salpingo oophorectomy
splenectomy
tendoplasty
thoracotomy
trabeculoplasty
ureterocystostomy
valvuloplasty
ventriculoperitoneal shunt

➤ RESOURCE CATEGORY 3:
WORD ROOTS, PREFIXES, AND SUFFIXES

Word Roots

Note: These are listed in their combining form.

abdomin/o
arthr/o
cardi/o
colon/o
crani/o
cutane/o
cyst/o
cyt/o
derm/o
enter/o
gastr/o
hemat/o
hepat/o
hyster/o
lith/o

muscul/o
my/o
neph/ro
neur/o
oophor/o
orchid/o
oste/o
phleb/o
rhin/o
therm/o
thorac/o
troph/o
tympan/o
ventr/o
vesic/o

Prefixes

ab-
ad-
allo-
an-
apo-
auto-
brachy-
brady-
contra-
dis-
dys-
ec-
ecto-
endo-
epi-

eu-
heme-
hyper-
hypo-
infra-
intra-
iso-
macro-
neo-
oto-
pan-
per-
supra-
tachy-
xeno-

Suffixes

-al
-ase
-asthenia
-ate
-blast
-cele
-centesis
-cephalus
-cle
-derma
-desis
-dynia
-eal
-ectasis
-ectomy

-emia
-entery
–gravida
-ic
-ism
-itis
-lith
-lysis
-ole
-oma
-phil
-plasia
-plasty
-rrhaphy
-rrhea

Medical Abbreviations

3

> ## COMMON MEDICAL ABBREVIATIONS

ABC   airway, breathing, circulation
abd.   abdomen
ABG   arterial blood gas
ABO   system of classifying blood groups
ac   before meals
ACE   angiotensin converting enzyme
ACS   acute compartment syndrome
ACTH   adrenocorticotrophic hormone
ADH   antidiuretic hormone
ADL   activities of daily living
ad lib   freely, as desired
AFP   alpha-fetoprotein
AIDS   acquired immunodeficiency syndrome
AKA   above the knee amputation
ALL   acute lymphocytic leukemia
ALS   amyotrophic lateral sclerosis
ALT   alkaline phosphatase (formerly SGPT)
AMI   antibody-mediated immunity
AML   acute myelogenous leukemia
amt.   amount
ANA   antinuclear antibody
ANS   autonomic nervous system
AP   anteroposterior
A&P   anterior and posterior

APC   atrial premature contraction
aq.   water
ARDS   adult respiratory distress syndrome
ASD   atrial septal defect
ASHD   atherosclerotic heart disease
AST   aspartate aminotransferase (formerly SGOT)
ATP   adenosine triphosphate
AV   atrioventricular
BCG   Bacille Calmette-Guerin
bid   two times a day
BKA   below the knee amputation
BLS   basic life support
BMR   basal metabolic rate
BP   blood pressure
BPH   benign prostatic hypertrophy
bpm   beats per minute
BPR   bathroom privileges
BSA   body surface area
BUN   blood, urea, nitrogen
C   centigrade, Celsius
c̄   with
Ca   calcium
CA   cancer
CABG   coronary artery bypass graft
CAD   coronary artery disease
CAPD   continuous ambulatory peritoneal dialysis
caps   capsules
CBC   complete blood count
CC   chief complaint
CCU   coronary care unit, critical care unit
CDC   Centers for Disease Control and Prevention
CHF   congestive heart failure
CK   creatine kinase
Cl   chloride
CLL   chronic lymphocytic leukemia
cm   centimeter
CMV   cytomegalovirus infection

CNS	central nervous system
CO	carbon monoxide, cardiac output
CO₂	carbon dioxide
comp	compound
cont	continuous
COPD	chronic obstructive pulmonary disease
CP	cerebral palsy
CPAP	continuous positive airway pressure
CPK	creatine phosphokinase
CPR	cardiopulmonary resuscitation
CRP	C-reactive protein
C&S	culture and sensitivity
CSF	cerebrospinal fluid
CT	computerized tomography
CTD	connective tissue disease
CTS	carpal tunnel syndrome
cu	cubic
CVA	cerebrovascular accident or costovertebral angle
CVC	central venous catheter
CVP	central venous pressure
DC	discontinue
D&C	dilation and curettage
DIC	disseminated intravascular coagulation
DIFF	differential blood count
dil.	dilute
DJD	degenerative joint disease
DKA	diabetic ketoacidosis
dl	deciliter (100 ml)
DM	diabetes mellitus
DNA	deoxyribonucleic acid
DNR	do not resuscitate
DO	doctor of osteopathy
DOE	dyspnea on exertion
DPT	vaccine for diphtheria, pertussis, tetanus
Dr.	doctor
DVT	deep vein thrombosis
D/W	dextrose in water

Dx   diagnosis
ECF   extracellular fluid
ECG or **EKG**   electrocardiogram
ECT   electroconvulsive therapy
ED   emergency department
EEG   electroencephalogram
EMD   electromechanical dissociation
EMG   electromyography
ENT   ear, nose, and throat
ESR   erythrocyte sedimentation rate
ESRD   end stage renal disease
ET   endotracheal tube
F   Fahrenheit
FBD   fibrocystic breast disease
FBS   fasting blood sugar
FDA   Food and Drug Administration
FFP   fresh frozen plasma
fl   fluid
4 x 4   piece of gauze 4" by 4" used for dressings
FSH   follicle-stimulating hormone
ft.   foot, feet (unit of measure)
FUO   fever of undetermined origin
g, gm   gram
GB   gallbladder
GFR   glomerular filtration rate
GH   growth hormone
GI   gastrointestinal
gr   grain
GSC   Glasgow coma scale
gtts   drops
GU   genitourinary
GYN   gynecological
h or **hrs**   hour or hours
(H)   hypodermically
Hb or **Hgb**   hemoglobin
HCG   human chorionic gonadotropin
HCO$_3$–   bicarbonate

Hct	hematocrit
HD	hemodialysis
HDL	high-density lipoproteins
Hg	mercury
Hgb	hemoglobin
HGH	human growth hormone
HHNC	hyperglycemia hyperosmolar nonketotic coma
HIV	human immunodeficiency virus
HLA	human leukocyte antigen
HR	heart rate
hr	hour
HSV	herpes simplex virus
HTN	hypertension
H_2O	water
Hx	history
Hz	hertz (cycles/second)
IAPB	intra-aortic balloon pump
IBBP	intermittent positive pressure breathing
IBS	irritable bowel syndrome
ICF	intracellular fluid
ICP	increased intracranial pressure
ICS	intercostal space
ICU	intensive care unit
IDDM	insulin dependent diabetes mellitus
IgA	immunoglobulin A
IM	intramuscular
I&O	intake and output
IOP	increased intraocular pressure
IPG	impedance plethysmogram
IPPB	intermittent positive-pressure breathing
IUD	intrauterine device
IV	intravenous
IVC	intraventricular catheter
IVP	intravenous pyelogram
JRA	juvenile rheumatoid arthritis
K^+	potassium
kcal	kilocalorie (food calorie)

kg kilogram
KO, KVO keep vein open
KS Kaposi's sarcoma
KUB kidneys, ureters, bladder
L, l liter
lab laboratory
lb. pound
LBBB left bundle branch block
LDH lactate dehydrogenase
LDL low-density lipoproteins
LE lupus erythematosus
LH luteinizing hormone
liq liquid
LLQ left lower quadrant
LOC level of consciousness
LP lumbar puncture
LPN, LVN licensed practical or vocational nurse
Lt, lt left
LTC long term care
LUQ left upper quadrant
LV left ventricle
m minum, meter, micron
MAO monoamine oxidase inhibitors
MAST military antishock trousers
mcg microgram
MCH mean corpuscular hemoglobin
MCV mean corpuscular volume
MD muscular dystrophy, medical doctor
MDI metered dose inhaler
mEq milliequivalent
mg milligram
Mg magnesium
MG myasthenia gravis
MI myocardial infarction
ml milliliter
mm millimeter
MMR vaccine for measles, mumps, rubella

MRI magnetic resonance imaging

MS multiple sclerosis

N nitrogen, normal (strength of solution)

NIDDM non-insulin dependent diabetes mellitus

Na+ sodium

NaCl sodium chloride

NANDA North American Nursing Diagnosis Association

NG nasogastric

NGT nasogastric tube

NLN National League for Nursing

noc at night

NPO nothing by mouth

NS normal saline

NSAIDS nonsteroidal anti-inflammatory drugs

NSNA National Student Nurses' Association

NST non-stress test

O_2 oxygen

OB-GYN obstetrics and gynecology

OCT oxytocin challenge test

OOB out of bed

OPC outpatient clinic

OR operating room

$\overline{os}$ by mouth

OSHA Occupational Safety and Health Administration

OTC over the counter (drug that can be obtained without a prescription)

oz. ounce

$\overline{p}$ with

P pulse, pressure, phosphorus

PA Chest posterior-anterior chest x-ray

PAC premature atrial complexes

$PaCO_2$ partial pressure of carbon dioxide in arterial blood

PaO_2 partial pressure of oxygen in arterial blood

PAD peripheral artery disease

Pap Papanicolaou smear

pc after meals

PCA patient controlled analgesia

PCO₂ partial pressure of carbon dioxide

PCP Pneumocystis carinii pneumonia

PD peritoneal dialysis

PE pulmonary embolism

PEEP positive end-expiratory pressure

PERRLA pupils equal, round, react to light and accommodation

PET postural emission tomography

PFT pulmonary function tests

pH hydrogen ion concentration

PID pelvic inflammatory disease

PKD polycystic disease

PKU phenylketonuria

PMS premenstrual syndrome

PND paroxysmal nocturnal dyspnea

PO, po by mouth

PO₂ partial pressure of oxygen

PPD positive purified protein derivative (of tuberculin)

PPN partial parenteral nutrition

PRN, prn as needed, whenever necessary

pro time prothrombin time

PSA prostate-specific antigen

psi pounds per square inch

PSP phenol-sulfonphthalein

PT physical therapy, prothrombin time

PTCA percutaneous transluminal coronary angioplasty

PTH parathyroid hormone

PTT partial thromboplastin time

PUD peptic ulcer disease

PVC premature ventricular contraction

q every

QA quality assurance

qh every hour

q 2 h every two hours

q 4 h every four hours

qid four times a day

qs quantity sufficient

R   rectal temperature, respirations, roentgen
RA   rheumatoid arthritis
RAI radioactive iodine
RAIU radioactive iodine uptake
RAS reticular activating system
RBBB right bundle branch block
RBC red blood cell or count
RCA right coronary artery
RDA recommended dietary allowance
resp respirations
RF   rheumatic fever, rheumatoid factor
Rh   antigen on blood cell indicated by + or –
RIND reversible ischemic neurologic deficit
RLQ right lower quadrant
RN   registered nurse
RNA ribonucleic acid
R/O, r/o rule out, to exclude
ROM range of motion (of joint)
Rt, rt right
RUQ right upper quadrant
Rx   prescription
s̄   without
S. or Sig.   (Signa) to write on label
SA   sinoatrial node
SaO2 systemic arterial oxygen saturation (%)
sat sol saturated solution
SBE subacute bacterial endocarditis
SDA same day admission
SDS same day surgery
sed rate sedimentation rate
SGOT serum glutamic-oxaloacetic transaminase (see AST)
SGPT serum glutamic-pyruvic transaminase (see ALT)
SI   International System of Units
SIADH syndrome of inappropriate antidiuretic hormone
SIDS sudden infant death syndrome
SL   sublingual
SLE systemic lupus erythematosus

SOB   short of breath
sol   solution
SMBG   self-monitoring blood glucose
SMR   submucous resection
sp gr   specific gravity
spec.   specimen
$\overline{ss}$ one half
SS   soap suds
SSKI   saturated solution of potassium iodide
stat   immediately
STD   sexually transmitted disease
subcut   subcutaneous
sx   symptoms
Syr.   syrup
T   temperature, thoracic to be followed by the number
      designating specific thoracic vertebra
T&A   tonsillectomy and adenoidectomy
tabs   tablets
TB   tuberculosis
T&C   type and crossmatch
TED   antiembolitic stockings
temp   temperature
TENS   transcutaneous electrical nerve stimulation
TIA   transient ischemic attack
TIBC   total iron binding capacity
tid   three times a day
tinct, or **tr.**   tincture
TMJ   temporomandibular joint
t-pa, TPA   tissue plasminogen activator
TPN   total parenteral nutrition
TPR   temperature, pulse, respiration
TQM   total quality management
TSE   testicular self-examination
TSH   thyroid-stimulating hormone
tsp   teaspoon
TSS   toxic shock syndrome
TURP   transurethral prostatectomy

UA   urinalysis
ung   ointment
URI   upper respiratory tract infection
UTI   urinary tract infection
VAD   venous access device
VDRL   Veneral Disease Research laboratory (test for syphilis)
VF, Vfib   ventricular fibrillation
VPC   ventricular premature complexes
VS, vs   vital signs
VSD   ventricular septal defect
VT   ventricular tachycardia
WBC   white blood cell or count
WHO   World Health Organization
wt   weight

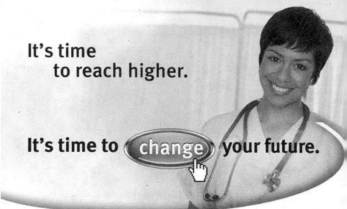